PRAISES FOR BREATHE, REPEAT

"This might be too cliché but it is appropriate — Breath, Repeat is a breath of fresh air to the self-help healing sector. I particularly liked Vincent's no-fluff, pragmatic guidance on how to heal our body and mind. The exercises are super easy, and I can attest, very effective. I highly recommend this book."

Paul Rodney Turner, The Food Yogi

"Essential instruction for optimizing brain health and function through the science and art of meditation. Vincent is a gifted guide, and in this book, he generously opens the door to put you on the journey of mastering breath work and meditation."

Dr. Sakib S. Qureshi, MD, Neurologist

BREATHE, REPEAT

A Busy Person's Guide to Preventing
Burn-out, Building Resilience and
Conquering Anxiety

VINCENT HU, CHC

DEDICATION

To my mom, who braved 8,000 miles with nothing but sheer determination and love.

To Karolina, who always believed in me.

To David Fink, whom I never met but whose book saved my life!

CONTENT

1. Introduction   1

2. My Story   5

3. Brain Basics: Understanding the Brain –
    Conditioning and Auto-Responses   14

4. Getting Unstuck:
    Tips and Tricks to Get Unstuck Fast   19

5. Breathe Like Your Life Depends On It:
    Build Resilience One Breath at a Time   36

6. Chill Out & Calm Down:
    Conquer Anxiety with Muscle Relaxation   64

7. Emotional Release: Letting Go and Surrendering   79

8. Putting It All Together:
    The 21-Day Challenge and Beyond   101

9. The Journey Continues   115

References   118

About Vincent   122

Acknowledgement   123

1

INTRODUCTION

Start Small to See Big Changes

The pace of modern life is exhausting. We all feel it. We find ourselves swept up in a nonstop whirlwind of stress and activity: constantly checking our email, glancing at our phones even when there's no text to answer, running around like time is a race — and the only way to win is to do things faster, quicker and more efficiently than everyone else around us. But exhaustion isn't what life is about.

Stress is normal, yes, but it doesn't have to control your life. You have the power to become the master of stress rather than its puppet. The exercises in this book are designed to help you reduce and manage the stresses of your daily life.

We've all read a million articles, books and life hacks about how to be more productive and get more done during the day...but to what end? What do we really want to accomplish in our lives? What are the things that really bring us joy, satisfaction, peace and happiness?

The best way to change your stress-filled, anxiety-ridden life isn't by reading about more productivity tricks or adding more life hacks to your already busy day. Deep down, you probably already know this. Doing more-more-more all the time is not the solution.

This book won't teach you how to get 8 hours of work done in half the time. It won't teach you how to create detailed to-do lists. It won't teach you how to become more organized, either, although you may become that way as a result of learning these methods.

This book *will* teach you a new way of life, one that will truly make you feel happier, more relaxed and more peaceful. And you don't have to make any big purchases or sign up for an expensive online course to do it.

Breathe, Repeat will help you de-stress and create more valuable free time in your daily life. This book will also provide you with easy strategies to feel more at ease throughout the day by guiding you through a deeper understanding of how breathing techniques, meditation and other relaxation methods are the backbone of living a centered, purposeful and meaningful life.

Most of what you read about productivity hacks, stress relievers and tips for staying organized don't get to the core of the problem. These so-called tricks and tips are the nails in your toolbox, but what you really need are hammers. Even if you only use some of them, the tools in *Breathe, Repeat* will give you what you really need to change your life.

We've all heard the phrase "change is hard," and for most people, that's true — many of us struggle to make even small changes to our daily lives. That's because we've been thinking about it all wrong this whole time. Instead of trying to make change easy, we simply need to allow change to happen. After reading this book, you'll know exactly what I mean when I talk about *allowing* change as opposed to trying to *force* change.

2

MY STORY

From Being Stressed, Afraid and Anxious to Calm, Zen and Grounded

This book was written by a software engineer who was once like you: I was stressed out, filled with anxiety and often overwhelmed by the big and small tasks of daily life. When I was a child, I would wake up in the morning already worried about the day. Anxiety was normal thing for me.

As a shy, introverted and anxious kid raised by a single mom living in a low income area of Washington, DC, I spent most of my life believing that working hard and putting in long hours was the only way to be successful. For many of us, getting top grades and doing well in school when we were younger meant that we would get a good job after college, which would equal a happy life filled with prosperity.

In all my years of schooling, though, I never stopped to consider the bigger picture. As kids, many of us were taught that work — whether it be schoolwork or our jobs — was the most important aspect of our lives. However, as we go through the trials and struggles of adulthood, we realize that finding true happiness is so much more complicated than doing a good job at school or work...or at least, it feels that way.

During my college years, I experienced a long period of depression, self-loathing and loneliness. The pressure-cooker environment of academic life was getting to me. My grades plummeted, and I had very few friends. For the last 2 years of college, I lived a very secluded life, using TV shows, movies and games to distract myself from my problems. I constantly had suicidal thoughts and even considered ending my life. I was also a sugarholic, downing can after can of

Mountain Dew, bottle after bottle of Sprite and bar after bar of Snickers. Little did I know that sugar was causing much of my anxiety and depression.

At first, I sought help by talking to a college counselor. Seeing a counselor helped tremendously — counseling sessions gave me a safe space to share the thoughts and feelings I had kept bottled up inside all those years.

Thanks to my counselor, I learned one of the biggest lessons in life: it's OK to fail. I actually had to practice "failing" and letting go of the need to be perfect. I had always felt pressured to get perfect grades, but thanks to my counselor, I realized this was a pressure I had put on myself.

For the first time in my life, I gave myself permission to fail — and I did. During my junior year of college, I received my first "F" ever. In the past, this scenario would have been my worst nightmare. But when it actually happened, in a way, failing was a relief. The burden to be perfect was lifted and I no longer cared so much. With my counselor's support and recommendation, I took six months off from school.

During my time off, I randomly came across a book called Release from Nervous Tension at my local library. The author, David Fink, recommended relaxation exercises to combat insomnia and anxiety. I began practicing self-directed muscle relaxation and experimented with deep breathing exercises on my own. This was the first time I became aware of involuntary tension in my gut when I was in unfamiliar social situations.

After 3 months of daily practice, I started to notice a huge shift: I had an abundance of energy and vitality. After 6 months of practice, I found myself totally transformed. At the age of 19, I went from being a shy, introverted kid who always wanted to retreat from the world to being a fearless extrovert.

I greeted everyone I met on the street. I talked to strangers on the subway in NYC and DC. I found myself sharing my feelings and speaking honestly with my mother and sister (which in Chinese and Asian cultures is a VERY difficult thing to do). I didn't know it at the time, but I had started to tap into the unconditional love that was already inside me, a love that had been buried by many years of depression, anxiety and living in fear. I felt more compassion towards others and I received more kindness in return.

With my new way of being, I had the confidence and energy to return to college and finish my degree. I also started to eat better, ditching sugar and switching to a vegetarian diet. I started doing yoga and began reading self-help books about psychology, holistic health and spiritual topics. I realized that so many of the medical issues I had had — ulcers, ADD/ADHD, hypoglycemia, a barrage of prescriptions for antibiotics — had been the result of my stressed-out, fearful lifestyle.

Five years later, I continued my studies by training with master teachers in holistic nutrition, meditation and yoga. I became certified as a health coach and yoga instructor and started coaching busy professionals, entrepreneurs and executives on the importance of healthy eating and living a balanced lifestyle. I taught meditation and breathing workshops to corporations and government agencies. I was proud to work with a team of health coaches at the National Integrated Health Associates in Washington, DC, the leading integrated medical practice on the East Coast. We helped them create the first nutrition and lifestyle program at their medical center.

The Lost Manual

Most of us are never given a manual on how to operate the human body. Like our parents and their parents, we navigate through life like conditioned creatures who are doomed to repeat our parents' bad habits and coping mechanisms.

Breathe, Repeat is a collection of over 25 years of my best health tips, tricks and biohacks that will allow you to break away from old habits that no longer serve you. It is the lost manual that will help you unlock the human potential within yourself.

In *Breathe, Repeat*, I've laid out a 21-day mindfulness and breathwork program for beginners. All of the breathing exercises in this book are backed by the latest research on yoga and meditation, giving you the opportunity to learn new ways to breathe like you never have before. There are exercises designed for experienced meditators, too.

Once you're ready for the next stage of my process, you can immerse yourself in the 30-day relaxation program in Chapter 6. This program is a modified and upgraded version of the original relaxation technique I used, the one that took me 3 to 6 months to get results. Now that I've refined the technique, within 3 to 4 weeks of doing the techniques and exercises in Chapter 6, you will feel more relaxed, calm and centered. I will teach you how to develop your muscle memory so that rather than tensing up during stressful situations, you'll be able to relax your body.

Power to Change

We all have the power to change, yet our old habits and self-limiting thoughts get in the way of this and keep us comfortable with the status quo. Let's get real: comfort is easy, while change can be difficult. For many of us, change can create fear and anxiety and bring up a slew of intense emotions. It's easier to binge on Netflix, food or alcohol to numb the pain. Change requires work. We have enough work on our plates already — why work on change, too?

The answer lies on what's on the other side of change: aliveness, freedom, growth, an abundance of energy and many other benefits. This is a story of my personal transformation, one that I'm hoping can serve as a blueprint and inspiration for others. As I'm writing this, I'm creating the change I want to see in the world. I want to share my story with those who are feeling stuck and afraid of change but are ready to take action.

The reality is this: change is a constant in our lives. If you are not growing, then you are withering. Change forces us to keep reaching forward towards our heart's desires, much like a sunflower reaching for the sun.

Our heart has an inner GPS that knows its true north. Change is the vehicle that brings us closer to our goals, our dreams, our truth and our union with GOD or whatever your spiritual inclination is for the unknown creator of this multi-verse.

Let's begin the journey now. Let's take a breath in, then exhale. And then repeat.

How to Use this Book: A Few Simple Tips

1. *Start small and go slow.* This is exactly what this book is intended to help you practice. Begin with the basic techniques and work your way up to the more challenging ones.

2. *Focus on building systems.* Begin with one or two daily practices. This will allow you to develop your breathing and relaxation techniques, which in turn will make it easier to adopt the other exercises. It is better to master one daily practice than to have a half-hearted understanding of a dozen.

3. *Set yourself up for success.* Make an intention to change today. To engage in the exercises in this book, it's best to commit yourself fully. Set up a regular time to do these techniques, have a timer on hand, create a designated space in your home for your practice, and

get support (like an online forum) to motivate you to keep going.

4. *Get pumped!* You are about to feel more cool, calm and collected in all areas of your life, and you won't even have to become a full-fledged Zen or meditation master to gain newfound bliss.

3

BRAIN BASICS

Understanding the Brain —
Conditioning and Auto-Responses

We tend to think of the brain like a machine, comprised of individual parts that have a specific function and operate exactly the way they are designed to. This is helpful for getting a general idea of how the brain works, but it isn't the whole picture. Unlike a machine, the brain is a complex organ, and it responds differently depending on certain conditions or circumstances.

Research has demonstrated that our environment and thoughts can physically alter our brain and thus our emotional responses.[1] Over time, our brain becomes conditioned to these responses, to the point where they feel automatic. For example, when you first start learning how to drive, your brain forms new neural pathways. These pathways produce a physical or mental response. This is why, when you see a red stop sign, you immediately think "Stop!" or you put your foot on the brake. Your brain associates the color red and the octagonal shape of the stop sign with a specific physical response.

The brain also forms neural pathways as you learn and practice emotional skills. Your emotional responses to experiences are the result of well-worn neural pathways you develop over your lifetime. Let's get back to driving and talk about an experience we've all had: getting stuck in traffic. For many of us, when we are stuck or waiting in traffic, our automatic response is to feel angry, frustrated or annoyed. We're conscious of feeling that way. Unconsciously, however, here's how the brain processes these feelings: whenever we get angry when we are in traffic, we strengthen the neural pathway that associates traffic with a negative emotion.

What if instead of honking the horn or cursing the car ahead of us every time we get stuck in a traffic jam, we were to practice feeling calm and relaxed? Over time, the neural pathways in our brain would start to associate traffic with peace and stillness. After all, by feeling angry every time we are in traffic, we are strengthening a neural pathway associated with negativity and cementing that emotional response. Wouldn't it be great to feel positive emotions instead?

To do this, we need to observe the negative emotions we are feeling in that moment and then try practicing a different emotional response. At first this is difficult, because we already have a well-developed neural pathway that links traffic with anger. But by consciously inhibiting this pathway, we help unwire these connections and strengthen a different response.

By adopting one or all three of the daily habits mentioned in this book, you can train yourself to notice your negative emotional responses and train yourself to react differently. As we practice responding to annoying or frustrating traffic situations with peace, we develop a new neural pathway; as that pathway is used more and more, it becomes easier for our brains to choose more positive emotions.

While it's true that our genes influence our temperament, we actually have more control over our minds than many of us realize. Our mental state directly affects our emotions — if we want to feel and experience more happiness, patience, tolerance, compassion and kindness in our lives, we have the power to do so.

When we are more relaxed and less stressed, we become more conscious of these negative auto-responses. Breathing and other relaxation techniques can help you develop new, more positive mental patterns more easily.

We can build new neural pathways in our brains and dampen the ones associated with anxiety, stress, fear and anger. Remember when you were first learning how to drive? It took more work to pay attention to all that was going on both inside and outside the car. Re-conditioning your brain is the same way. At first, you will have to pay closer attention to what's going on in your own thoughts, and you may feel uncomfortable doing some of these exercises. But know that you are now in the driver's seat of your own mind. Soon you will be well on your way to feeling more calm, relaxed and serene — even in traffic!

The rest of this book will help you become more flexible with your responses to daily stressors. These daily relaxation and breathing exercises will help loosen the narrow perceptions of life that many of us have become accustomed to, thereby allowing us to see more choices. Likewise, the mindfulness practices in the next chapters will allow you to unleash your grasp of old habits and open yourself up to new, more powerful ways of consciousness.

Are you ready to start building your new neural pathways?

4

GETTING UNSTUCK

Tips and Tricks to Get Unstuck Fast

Why do we worry? Think about it. Worry is different than fear, which is a natural response to a dangerous, threatening or alarming situation. In many ways, fear can be a good emotion — it tells us that we need to be cautious or look out for potential hazards. Let's say you're hiking along a mountain or hillside, but on one side there is a steep drop-off. To feel fear in this situation would be normal, as it alerts your body to the fact that you could fall and be seriously injured.

Now let's say you're walking along a flat path, with no cliff or drop-off on either side. And yet, during the walk, you're constantly worried about falling and breaking your ankle. This is the difference between fear and worry: one is a natural, normal response to an unsafe situation, while the other plagues our minds with unnecessary stress and anxiety.

Worrying is just one type of what I like to call "being stuck." Being stuck can refer to uncontrollable, repetitive thoughts that we can't seem to stop or manage. There is also the idea of being emotionally stuck, which includes worrying too much about things beyond our control.

Worry also relates to anxiety. Before an important test, it's normal to feel some type of stress. To combat this, you might spend a lot of time studying, or you might try to sleep well the night before. Once the test is over, you feel relieved and most of your stress subsides.

Anxiety is a different feeling. If you have a big test coming up and you're anxious, you may worry constantly, which would make it hard to focus while you're studying. During a test, an anxious person might feel nervous, sweaty or have uncontrollable thoughts. Then, even after the exam, an anxious person could still be wrapped up in their worries even though the stressful situation is over.

Fortunately, feelings of fear and anxiety don't have to be a daily occurrence. Over time, you've conditioned your brain to have these responses, but you can rewire your brain to have a different reaction to tense, stressful or high-pressure situations. The exercises and tips in this chapter will teach you how to get unstuck in a matter of minutes.

Our Physiology Affects Our Psychology

One of the quickest way to 'get unstuck' is by noticing how we hold ourselves in our body. When we slouch or hunch our backs, for example, our energy gets blocked, which makes us feel more sluggish and less confident. On the flip side, when we hold ourselves with our back straight and chest expanded, we instantly notice a difference in our energy and our mood.

Just as how we carry ourselves affects our mood, how we feel affects our body. When we are depressed, we tend to have significantly less physical energy. Depressed people want to sleep a lot, and when sleeping might crouch into a fetal position, signaling a need for the body to protect itself. When we are joyful, we feel energized both physically and mentally.

The next time you feel sad, depressed or anxious, notice how you're holding your posture. Just by being aware of how your body physically responds to certain situations can help you change how you feel in any given situation.

That said, for most of us, anxiety begins in the mind. Our modern world has turned us into cerebral, thought-focused creatures. As a result, many of us have become detached or ungrounded from our physical selves. But only by getting in touch with our bodies can we reduce anxiety and achieve a calmer mental state.

The following exercises are designed to help you "get grounded" and move your body as a way of combating stress and anxiety.

4.1 One Minute Increase Flexibility Exercise

Let's get started with a simple exercise that can increase your flexibility by 20-30% — and in less than a minute! This exercise will you give you a taste of how you can get immediate results by working with the body's energies.

Time: Less than a minute

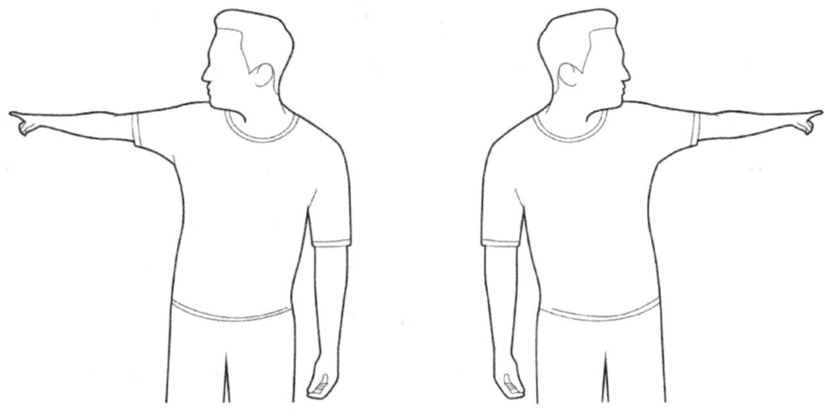

Figure 4.1.1

1. While standing, relax your arms by your sides.
2. Lift your right arm up until it's parallel to the floor.
3. While keeping your legs and head neutral, turn to the right from the waist and carry the arm around to the right.
4. Point your index finger at an object in front of you. This will be your starting point and a measure of how flexible you are right now (see figure 4.1.1). Remember that object, because we will use it again later.
5. Come back to center and relax your right arm.
6. Now let's do the same with your left arm and turn your left arm to the left and from the waist. Point to

an object and remember that location (see figure 4.1.1).

7. Come to center and start firmly rubbing your ears with your fingers firmly, massaging the inner lobes of your ears. You can tug on your ears as well.

8. Continue to rub your ears up and down your ears for 30-45 seconds. Some areas will feel more tender and tense than others.

9. Relax your arms for a few seconds and notice the heat and sensations around your ears.

10. Now do the first two exercises from the very beginning: point your right arm and index finger to the right and then to the left.

11. You should notice a difference and that you've gone farther with your twist/turn — you'll see that you're pointing at a different object.

Comments:

We are working with the acupuncture meridians along the ears, which shifts the energy in the body.

Getting Unstuck with Inversion

Yoga inversions are a great way to reset energy in the body. Inversions also give the heart a break — when you're upside down, the heart doesn't have to work as hard to get the blood to circulate back up from the legs since the normal pull of gravity is reversed.

4.2 Standing Inversion: Forward Bend

Here's a simple inversion you can do if you don't have the time or space to do a full head stand or shoulder stand.

Time: 1-3 minutes

1. Stand with your legs shoulder-width apart.
2. Fold forward while keeping your legs straight or slightly bent (see figure 4.2.1 below)
3. Allow your head, neck and arms to hang.
4. While inverted, breathe into your mouth, and drawing the air into your heart.
5. On the exhale, breathe out through your nose.
6. Practice this breath pattern for 3-5 minutes.
7. Slowly make your way back up. Notice any changes in energy, mood or focus.

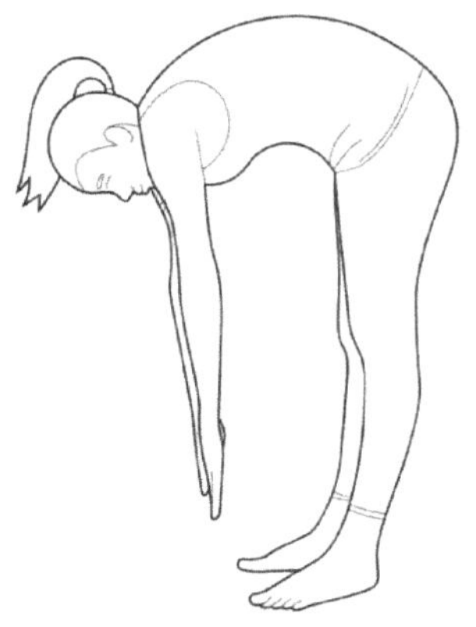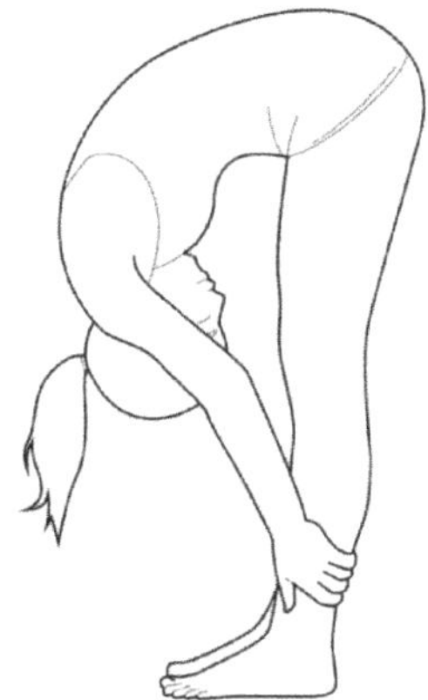

Figure 4.2.1

4.3 Get Unstuck with Your Partner

This is an exercise that you can do with your partner or a friend to help you "get unstuck' or diffuse any emotional upsets with the other person.

Time: 1-3 Minutes

1. Stand with legs wider than shoulder-width apart and with your back to the other person's back. Your backs should be 6 inches apart.
2. Fold forward (see figure 4.3.1) with both arms hanging by your sides.
3. Both of you close your eyes, and breathe in through the mouth and breathe out through the nose for 4-5 complete breaths.

4. Then slowly open eyes and gaze at each other between both of your sets of legs.

5. Bring up the issue or topic that you wanted to "get unstuck" from a few minutes ago. Notice if anything has shifted.

6. You or your partner may start to giggle or laugh at the other person because you are see each other in a different perspective.

7. After a minute or two, slowly rise up and face your partner. Again, notice if your perception of him/her has shifted. Begin to talk to each other about the experience.

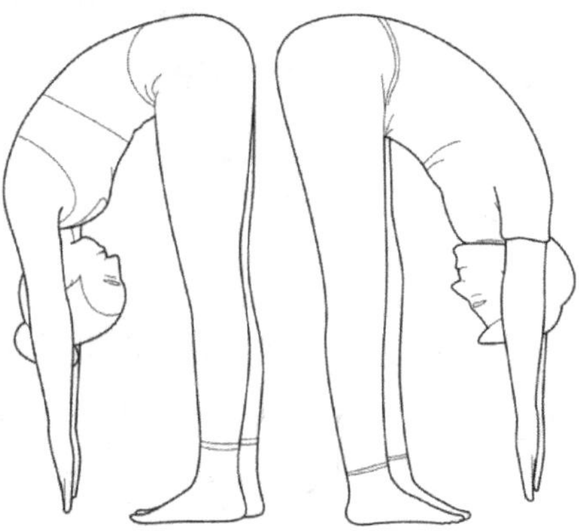

Figure 4.3.1

Getting Unstuck with Whole-Brain Integration

From time to time, the left (analytical) and right (creative) hemispheres of the brain get "hijacked" by our reptilian (animal) and limbic (emotional) brains.

Our reptilian and limbic brains are more ancient than the other parts of our brain — our brains have since evolved to become more rational and creative. The earliest humans, when faced with a "fight-or-flight" situation (like being chased by a predator) reacted by using their animal and emotional brains. There simply wasn't time to weigh the options (analytical) or brainstorm a new solution (creative) in these life-or-death situations.

In fearful or anxious situations, our animal and emotional brains still overtake our rational and emotional brains. Have you ever drawn a complete blank when asked to solve a math problem in front of an entire class? Public speaking is one of the best examples of this reaction — when placed in an uncomfortable situation like speaking in public, people often freeze. This is because when we sense fear, the reptilian part of our brain takes over and causes us to clam up.

Through many years of practice, I've discovered that the quickest and easiest way to prevent "freezing up" during a tense or stressful situation is by doing activities that target both the left and right hemispheres of the brain.

In a matter of minutes, the following exercises will help you focus, boost your creativity, improve your ability to think logically and increase your productivity throughout the day.

4.4 Whole Brain Exercise: March in Place (Cross Crawl)

Time: 1-2 minutes

1. Stand with your legs slightly apart.
2. Start marching in place (figure 4.4.1), with your left elbow crossing over your midline to the opposite side of your body as your right knee comes up to meet it.
3. Lift your left knee to touch your right elbow. Your left knee should cross over the midline of your body.
4. Continue the exaggerated march in place for up to minutes.

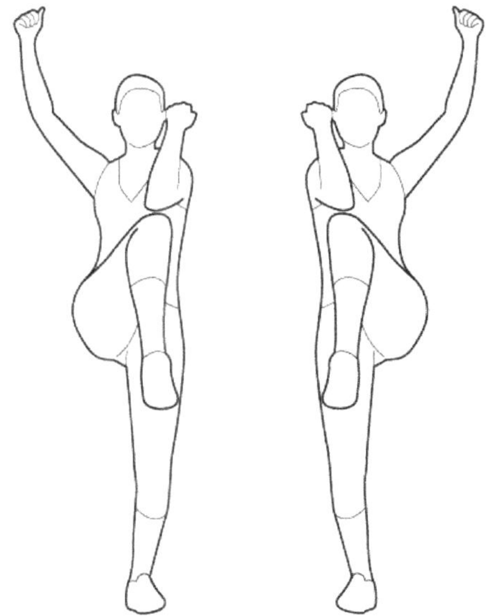

Figure 4.4.1

4.5 Whole Brain Exercise: Interlaced Fingers

Time: 1 minute

1. After marching in place, interlace your fingers together with your palms touching.
2. Breathe in through your mouth and out through your nose slowly and deeply.
3. Breathe and hold your palms together for 1 full minute.

4.6 Whole Brain Exercise: Eye Re-Focusing Exercise

Many of us spend a lot of time in front of a computer, which means we rarely focus our attention more than 2 to 3 feet away from our face. As a result, our muscles get locked into the same position for hours.

Borrowed from natural eye movement techniques, this exercise engages both the left and right hemispheres of the brain. Remember, the right brain is responsible for imagination and creativity, and left brain is responsible for order and logic (among other things).

Time: start with 1 minute and work up to 3 minutes.

1. Look at a single point that's more than 20 feet away and is directly in front of you. The farther away the point is, the better, so select an object in the distance. Focus only on a single point on that object (e.g., focus on the seat of a bicycle and not the whole bicycle).
2. Look at the tip of your nose and then shift your focus back out to the object you selected.
3. Do this 2-3 times: nose to object, object to nose.
4. Now, with your mind's eye, imagine a very long yellow pencil with a red eraser. Imagine that eraser is touching the tip of your nose, and the tip of the pencil is touching the object you selected in the distance.

5. Slowly shift your focus and attention from the eraser and along the yellow pencil, shifting your focus to the single point of the object in front of you.
6. Slowly bring your focus back from the selected object, tracing your way along the yellow pencil, and ending at tip of your nose/pencil's eraser.
7. Continue to focus, slowly shifting along the imaginary pencil for 1-3 minutes.
8. Breathe normally and consciously.

Comments:

It's important to select an object that's directly in front of you, right in your line of sight and at least 20 feet away.

If this your first time doing this exercise, you may notice some sensations around the muscles of your eyes.

When our brain is more integrated, with the left and right sides working together, we become more creative, focused and productive. These brain "workouts" were created for and first used with students who had trouble focusing on learning. Integrating your brain is one of the quickest ways to center yourself and focus on the task at hand.

Get Unstuck by Boosting Your Own Mood Levels

Recent studies have revealed that yoga stretches can naturally increase GABA levels in your brain. GABA (gamma-Aminobutyric acid) is an amino acid that primarily serves as a neurotransmitter. Neurotransmitters help your body function and regulate your moods, perceptions and sleep patterns. People with low GABA levels may experience depression, anxiety and insomnia. [1]

A 2007 Boston University School of Medicine found that practicing yoga can potentially elevate your GABA levels, thus alleviating symptoms of depression, anxiety and other mood disorders. [1]

If you're feeling out of balance or ungrounded, yoga poses and exercises — especially Hatha yoga — can help you regain that balance and feel centered again. Increasing your GABA levels has been shown to put you in a more relaxed state.

If you don't have time to go to a yoga class, you can do the following exercise.

4.7 Seated Forward Bend

Time: start with 2 minutes and work your way up to 5 minutes

1. Start by sitting on the floor with your legs in front of you. Keep your legs together, with your ankles touching and your feet flexed. Point your toes to the ceiling.
2. Raise your arms up to lengthen your spine, then exhale while bending forward from your hips.
3. Depending on your flexibility, grab any part of your legs that you can reach comfortably along your calves, or thighs or ankles. You can have a bend at your elbows if needed.
4. If you have tight hamstrings, you can add a slight bend in your knees for added comfort.
5. Allow your head and chest to rest on top of your thighs (or hover over them).
6. Breathe in deeply through your nose, as you expand your lower back.
7. Breathe out through your nose as you contract your belly inward, deepening the stretch even more.
8. Watch your breath flow in and out of your nose. Notice the coolness or warmth of your breath as you relax deeper into the pose.
9. For beginners, start with 2 minutes and work your way up to 10 minutes.

10. Transition out of this pose by lying on your back and hug your knees into your chest, rocking left and right a couple of times and relaxing your legs afterward.

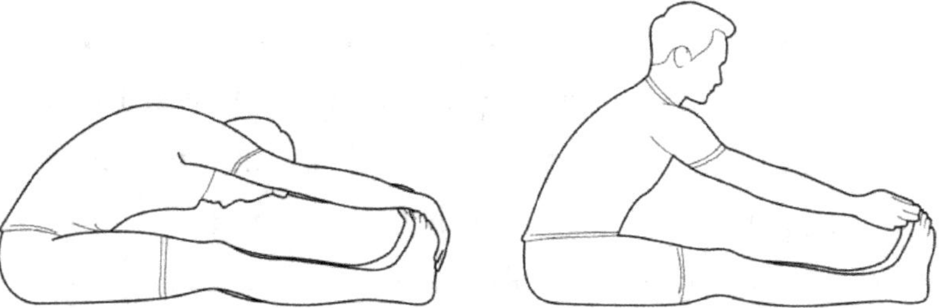

Figure 4.7.1

Comments:

It's important to remember to never force yourself into a stretch or to push too hard. Avoid any discomfort and never overstretch! Allow your body to relax into the position by doing deep breathing and mentally telling your tight muscles to "Relax and let go."

5

BREATHE LIKE YOUR LIFE DEPENDS ON IT

Build Resilience One Breath at a Time

Every moment of our lives, we are breathing…yet many of us never practice breathing or controlling our breath. You may think that you don't need to learn how to breathe — you're doing it right now without effort, right?

Yes, you are. However, learning to breathe properly when faced with stress is a key component of reducing your stress and going about your day in a relaxed, peaceful manner.

While breathing is innate, here's the truth: if you're feeling stressed, anxious or filled with worry, you're probably not breathing right. Breathing isn't just the process of inhaling oxygen and exhaling carbon dioxide — it also affects your emotions your mental state and your overall well-being.

Some stress can be beneficial at times. If you're studying for an exam or you're on a work deadline, stress can push you to prepare for the test or finish your project on time. However, an extreme amount of stress can have negative health consequences and adversely affect the immune, cardiovascular, neuroendocrine and central nervous systems.

According to the American Psychological Association (APA), chronic stress is linked to the six leading causes of death: heart disease, cancer, lung ailments, accidents, cirrhosis of the liver and suicide.[1] Roughly 60-80% of primary care visits may be related to stress — yet only 3% of patients receive stress management counseling.[1]

Unlike everyday stressors that can be managed with healthy stress management behaviors, untreated chronic stress can result in serious health conditions, including anxiety, insomnia, muscle pain, high blood pressure and a weakened immune system. Some studies have even suggested that unhealthy chronic stress management (such as overeating "comfort" foods) has contributed to the growing obesity epidemic. [1]

Despite the clear link between stress and illness, a recent APA Stress in America survey revealed that 33% of Americans never discuss ways to manage stress with their healthcare provider.[1]

Now, here's the good news: most stress-related diseases are preventable. One of the BEST tools to combat and manage chronic stress is to develop a Stress Reduction Breathing Practice (like the one in exercise 5.1).

By learning how to breathe right and take deeper breaths, you can greatly reduce stress and decrease your risk of serious health problems. This chapter will show you how to breathe like your life depends on it — because it does!

The Relaxation Response

Here's another piece of good news: while you can't control the stress response — it's automatic — or the stressors in your life, you can control the relaxation response.

Deep breathing exercises, muscle relaxation techniques and other Zen activities work because they activate the relaxation response. The term was first coined by Dr. Herbert Benson of Harvard Medical School as a scientific alternative to "meditation" — he used "relaxation response" to describe the ability of the body to stimulate the relaxation of muscles and organs.[2]

The relaxation response works like this: when we are stressed, we activate our body's sympathetic nervous system, which puts us in fight-or-flight mode. This state is meant to ready our bodies for intense physical activity. That backfires when we're stressed out all the time, because we get used to feeling like we're always in a high-pressure situation even when we're not.

However, when we meditate or engage in techniques that relax the body, we activate our parasympathetic nervous system, which puts us in a deep state of total relaxation.

The important thing to remember about the relaxation response is that we are in control, not our body. It's entirely possible to learn how to activate the parasympathetic nervous system to feel calmer and less tense in stressful situations.

5.1 The Anti-Stress Breathing Technique

Studies have shown that you can activate the relaxation response by changing your breath pattern. Here's a simple anti-stress breathing exercise to get you started on your way to a more stress-free life! This exercise can be done sitting or lying down, although if you're sitting, keep your spine straight as possible.

Time: set timer for 2 minutes. Build the practice up slowly to 5 minutes.

1. With your eyes closed, inhale deeply through your nose for a count of 4 seconds, filling your lungs to full capacity, but without causing any tension or pain.
2. Exhale through your mouth slowly and completely for a count of 8 seconds. Empty out the air from your lungs.
3. Let the exhale be longer than the inhale—if it takes

you 3 seconds to inhale, then take 6 seconds to exhale. You can lengthen your exhales by constricting your throat so that air takes longer to leave your lungs.

4. Repeat 1-3.

Comments:

Slow exhalation has a calming effect on the nervous system and the mind. This is a good exercise if you have trouble falling asleep or you have insomnia.

A Wandering Mind is an Unhappy Mind

For many of us, our minds wander frequently, regardless of what we're doing. Playing with smartphones, surfing the internet and other distractions have only made it harder for us to focus.

While we all get a little distracted sometimes, a wandering mind is an unhappy mind. In 2010, Harvard psychologists Matthew A. Killingsworth and Daniel T. Gilbert developed a special "Track Your Happiness" iPhone app to research people's ongoing thoughts, feelings and actions.[3] The researchers found that people are thinking about what is not happening in the moment almost as often as they are thinking about what is happening. Doing this typically made people unhappy,

Killingsworth and Gilbert found, leading the researchers to conclude that "A human mind is a wandering mind, and a wandering mind is an unhappy mind."[3]

Unlike other animals, human beings spend a lot of time thinking about things outside of the present moment: we contemplate events that happened in the past, what might happen in the future and even things that will never happen at all. Although this ability is a remarkable evolutionary achievement and one that enables us to learn, reason and plan ahead, it can come at an emotional cost.

Many philosophical and religious traditions teach that happiness is to be found by living in the moment — their practitioners are specifically trained to resist mind-wandering and "to be here now." These traditions also suggest that a wandering mind can be an unhappy mind.

The Mindful Breath

Contrary to popular belief, the purpose of meditation is not to quiet the mind — as the previously mentioned study shows, the main function of the mind is to think. It's perfectly normal to have thoughts while we're meditating or doing breathing exercises.

To further our goals, however, we can temporarily distract the mind with our breath. By activating the relaxation response or calming our nervous system, we can work to slow down our hyperactive "monkey mind."

Remember, our wandering mind is responding to stressors that either happened in past or have yet to occur in the future. Bringing our awareness back to the present — even momentarily at first — is a step along the pathway to greater happiness.

A few years back, I interviewed an experienced mindfulness meditation teacher about her practice. She shared this analogy about the "monkey mind":

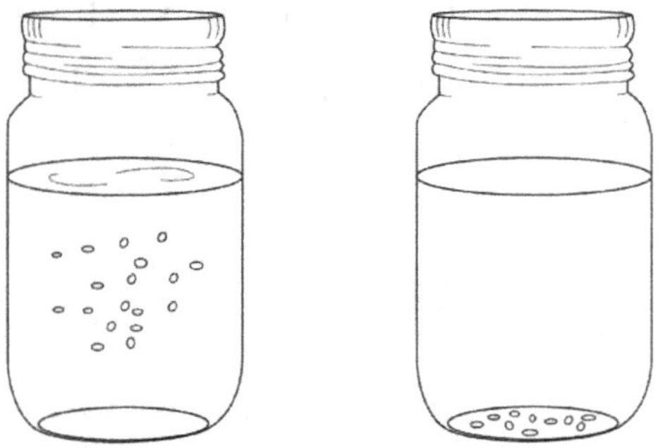

Figure 5.1.1

Imagine that your thoughts are like sugar or salt crystals, floating around in a glass of water after you give it a good stir (figure 5.1.1). These thoughts — which swirl around endlessly — will continue to move around your mind if you keep entertaining them.

However, by continuously practicing meditation and mindfulness, your thoughts will stop swirling and will settle to the bottom of the glass. By being present with your thoughts — not judging them, not pushing them away, or becoming too attached to them — eventually with time, they will settle down.

5.2 The Mindfulness Breathing Exercise

Here's a simple mindfulness exercise that help you stay present and get centered in matter of minutes.

Time: 2-5 minutes twice a day (or whenever you are feeling scattered and un-centered)

1. With your eyes closed, inhale through your nose for a count of 3-4 seconds (figure 5.2.1).
2. Notice if the air is cool or warm, fast or slow.
3. Notice if your nose is stuffed or clear.
4. As you exhale slowly for a count of 3-4 seconds, see if the exhalation is different from the inhalation (figure 5.2.1).
5. Notice if the inhale is easier to do than the exhale or

vice versa, or the same.

6. Pay attention to the texture, temperature or sensations of the exhalation.

7. Repeat steps 1 through 6, and just watch the breath flow in and out of nasal passage with all of your attention.

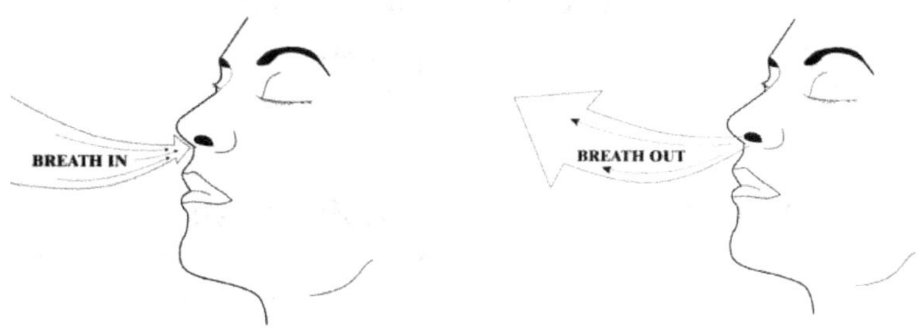

Figure 5.2.1

Comments:

This is a very simple and easy exercise to do, but it provides huge benefits. We are practicing being present in what is happening right now, without entertaining the thoughts of the future or the past. I find it extremely useful to practice this technique before engaging in any high-anxiety activities, like public speaking or confronting someone. It's a good reminder to your body that the fear you're about to face is not realistic and that the outcome is more often than not going to be better than you had expected.

Check in with yourself after the exercise. How did it go? How was your mind? Was it busy? That's normal. With practice, you can quickly bring yourself back into the present moment.

The Belly Breath

If you've ever taken a yoga class — or been dragged reluctantly by a friend, you've probably been told by the yoga teacher to "breathe deeply into your belly."

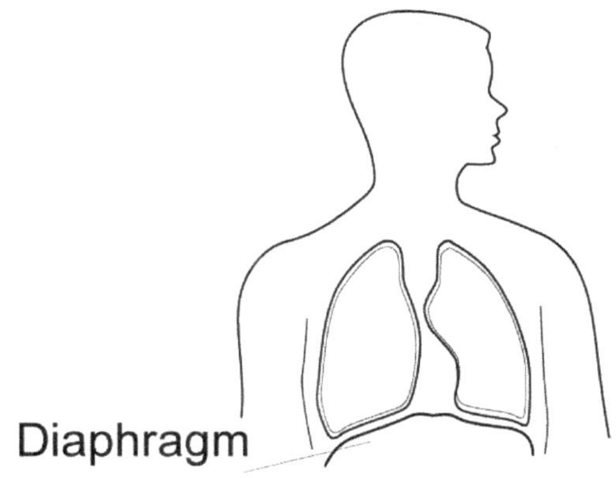

Figure 5.2.2

Belly breathing is an excellent way to lower your stress response. Belly breathing (also called diaphragmatic breathing or abdominal breathing) is something you can do anytime and anywhere. Belly breathing engages the diaphragm (figure 5.2.2), which is shaped like a parachute and consists of muscles and tendons that control our respiratory system and the breathing process.

Babies breathe from the diaphragm automatically—if you watch a sleeping baby, you'll notice that her belly rises up and down naturally. As people grow older, however, their stress increases, and they forget how to breathe from the belly. Instead, they start to breathe from the chest.

What Happens in Vagus

Deep belly breathing can significantly reduce the stress response. When you breathe deeply — from your diaphragm, not your chest — it's like you're stepping on a brake that stops stress in its tracks. That brake is called the vagus nerve.

The vagus nerve is the major nerve in the parasympathetic nervous system, the system that controls functions of the heart, lungs and digestive tract. When your sympathetic nervous system revs up your fight-or-flight response (pouring adrenaline and the stress hormone cortisol into your body at the same time), the vagus nerve is in charge of telling your body to "chill out" by releasing acetylcholine.

The vagus nerve is a voluntary nerve that can be strengthened. Some studies have revealed that people with a stronger vagus response may be more likely to recover quickly after injury, illness or moments of stress. In addition, a 2010 study published in *The Journal of Alternative and Complementary Medicine* showed that slow abdominal breaths (aka deep belly breathing) reduced the fight-or-flight response of the sympathetic nervous system.[4]

There are other benefits of stimulating the vagus nerve, including:

- Better cognitive function
- Increased psychological and physical resilience
- Reduced hypertension[4]
- Decreased anxiety[5]
- Lower inflammation[5]
- Improved memory[6]
- Could help you live longer[8]

Deep breathing is an extremely helpful technique for dealing with stressful situations. For example, I practice deep belly breathing whenever I have to deal with painful dental procedures, like tooth extractions or cavity fillings. Because of these deep belly breathing exercises, my pain tolerance is now very high these days.

I used to get overly anxious about deadlines at work — I felt like it was a matter of life or death if I didn't complete a project on time. Now, although I still feel some stress and anxiety, I'm able to manage it better, and it doesn't keep me up at night. Because I practice stress management, my resilience against and tolerance for stress is higher. During the weeks leading up to a deadline, I can now get through 10 to 12-hour workdays on only 5 or 6 hours of sleep without burning out. That's all due to my stress management practice.

Stress management, breathing techniques and meditation are also a great way to stay centered. No matter how stressed your life is, or how busy your "monkey mind" gets, you can always return to peace and stillness.

5.3 Belly Breathing (Diaphragmatic Breath for Beginners)

Belly breathing is done lying down or sitting down. For beginners, it's best to practice a few times while lying down—your diaphragms is less constricted this way.

5.3.1 Lying Down Practice

Time: 3-5 minutes

1. Lie on a flat surface or bed, with your legs shoulder-width apart. You can support your head with a pillow if you like.
2. With your eyes closed, inhale slowly through your nose for a count of 4 seconds.
3. As you inhale, imagine a balloon expanding around your belly, with your belly pushing out first on the inhalation (step 1 in figure 5.3.1)
4. Imagine the balloon expanding to the side of your rib cage, while simultaneously pushing outwards to the left and right of your rib cage.
5. Let the balloon continue to get bigger behind you, pressing your lower back towards the floor (step 2 in figure above).
6. Lastly, fill your lungs to full capacity without straining, expanding the balloon up towards your chest and collarbones (step 3 in figure 5.3.1 above).
7. At first, your lungs will feel tight. This is normal and expected since most people do not breathe deeply enough most of the time.
8. Exhale through your nose for a count of 8 seconds. Imagine that the balloon is deflating from the chest first, then pushing your belly in and up so that you can completely exhale all the air out of that balloon.

9. Repeat steps 1 through 8 for 3 to 5 minutes.

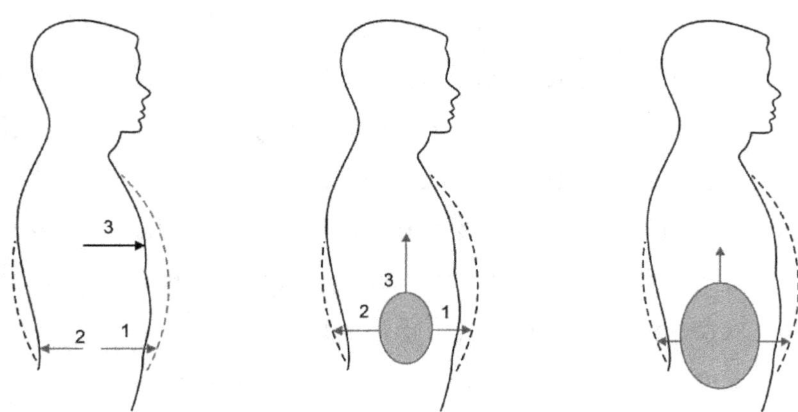

Figure 5.3.1

Comments:

If you're a beginner, you are working muscles you haven't used before or in a long time. Most of the clients I've seen who don't have a regular breathing practice have difficulty breathing from the belly. Start slow and never force your body to do anything it doesn't want to do. You can reduce the time it takes to inhale and exhale to 2-4 seconds.

<u>5.3.2 Sitting Practice</u>

Time: 3-5 minutes

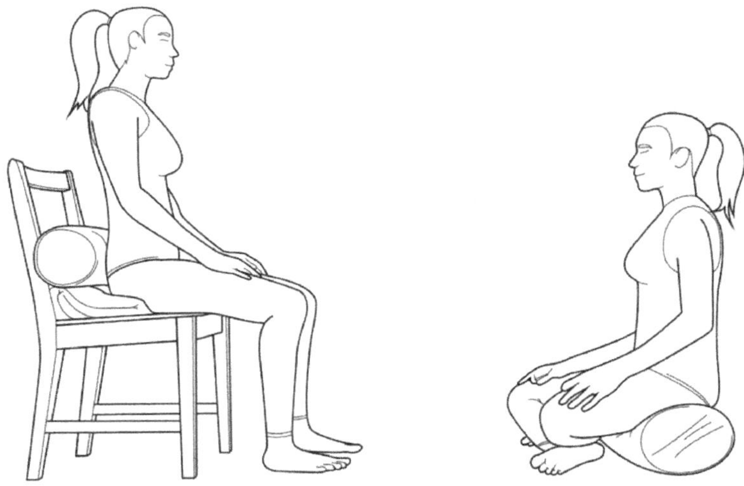

Figure 5.3.2a

1. Find a comfortable chair or sofa to sit on. Some people find it helpful to roll up a blanket (1-2 inches high) and

   put it under their buttocks to keep their back straight (see figure 5.3.2a). This also reduces strain on the hip area when sitting for a long period of time. If you're sitting on a chair, try to keep your feet flat on the floor and your back away from the backrest (people tend to slouch when their back touches the backrest). Your hands should be resting palm-up on tops of your knees and your arms should be relaxed.

2. With your eyes closed, breathe in slowly through your nose for a count of 4.
3. Imagine a balloon expanding below your belly (figure 5.3.2a), with your belly pushing out first.
4. Imagine the balloon expanding to the side of your rib cage while simultaneously pushing outwards to the left and right of your rib cage.
5. Expand the balloon towards to your lower back and mid-back (see step 2 in figure 5.3.2b).
6. Lastly, fill your lungs to full capacity, expanding the balloon up towards your chest and collarbone. Expand your chest outward.
7. Exhale for a count of 4 and imagine deflating the balloon from the chest first, then pushing your belly in and up so that you can completely exhale all the air out of the balloon.
8. Repeat steps 1 through 7.

Comments:

As you practice this technique, over time, the chest muscles around your lungs will begin to relax, allowing you to take in more air. Again, start slow and small to allow your body to get used to this new way of breathing.

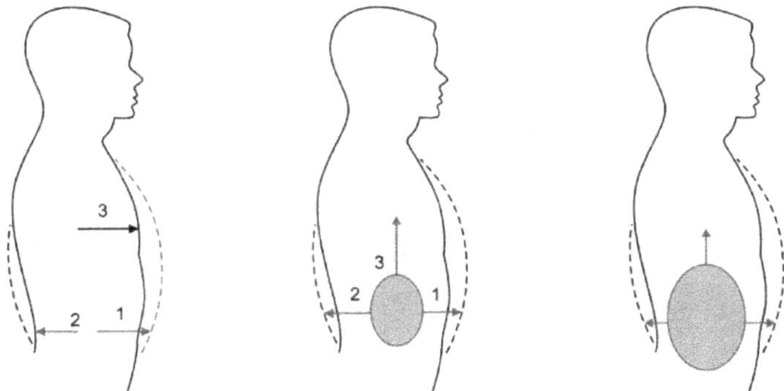

Figure 5.3.2b

5.4 The One-Minute Breath (Intermediate)

One exercise you can try is increasing the length of your inhalation and exhalation. Studies have shown that when people reduce their breath pattern to 6 breaths per minute, they have a higher heart rate variability, which is the time interval between heartbeats.[7] Multiple studies have revealed that a higher heart rate variability helps reduce stress and improve overall health.[7]

Time: 1 minute

1. With your eyes closed, inhale 5 small and equal sniffs through your nose, while expanding your belly and chest for a count of 5 seconds (about one sniff per

second). Make sure your belly and chest are relaxed when you inhale.

2. When you exhale, let out 5 small and equal sniffs through your nose for a count of 5 seconds. On the exhale, you can engage your belly by pushing the belly in and up towards your chest on each sniffle. This will take some time to get used to.

3. End by relaxing your breath and breathing normally.

Comments:

If done correctly, this exercise should take 10 seconds for a complete inhalation and exhalation (or 6 breaths per minute). This is a powerful breathing exercise that directly stimulates the vagus nerve and increases heart rate variability.

5.5 Pelvic Floor Breath for Ultra Zen (Advanced)

There's a reason why belly breathing is such a common command during yoga class: diaphragmatic breathing has a significant effect on your abdomen muscles and the pelvic floor, and breathing properly is important for the function of the pelvic floor. That's because your pelvic floor muscles need to stretch and contract. When you have poor posture (i.e., from being hunched over a computer all day), your abdomen muscles can become weak, which can also weaken your pelvic floor muscles.

This is why it's important to practice belly breathing — you want to keep your abdomen and pelvic floor muscles healthy and strong.

Time: 3-5 minutes.

Note: This exercise can be done lying down or sitting up.

1. Practice belly breathing (aka diaphragmatic breathing) for 2 minutes.
2. Inhale through your nose and expand your belly (steps 1 to 3, Figure 5.5.1), at the same time imagining a balloon filling up that's at the center of your belly (figure 5.5.1). Allow for space in your breath.
3. Imagine the balloon expanding behind your back and to the sides of your rib cage, filling your lungs to full capacity.

4. As you exhale through your nose, gently contract your lower abdomen, moving your navel toward your spine. Repeat a few times, each time emptying out the air more fully. As you inhale, let your belly relax and be soft. Allow the air to fill your lungs as your belly naturally inflates. Repeat for 3 to 5

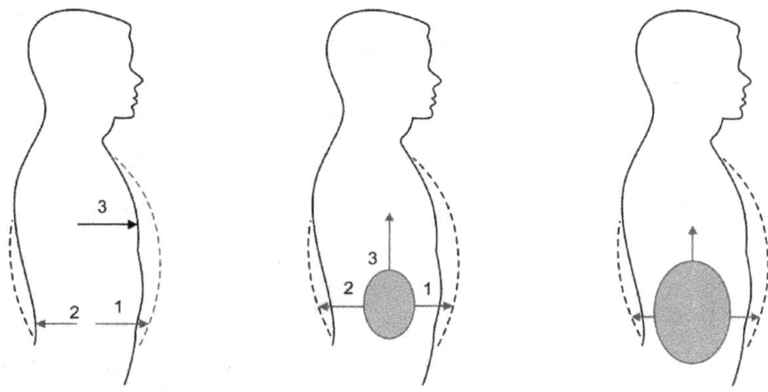

Figure 5.5.1

breaths, then just relax and return to your normal breath.

5. Relax for 1 minute.

6. Next, let's add an additional step to the belly breathing pattern.

7. On the next inhale, continue to use the balloon imagery and expand the balloon outwards (step 1 in figure 5.5.2), then expand the balloon downwards

toward your pelvic floor, which is located directly below your sex organs and at the perineum (step 2 in figure 5.5.2).

8. If done correctly, you should notice your internal organs (both the small and large intestine) press downwards slightly towards your perineum, which is the area between the anus and sex organs.

9. You don't physically move the breath or make contact with your perineum or pelvic floor — this is more of a visualization of an energetic contact or awareness that happens when you focus your attention on your pelvic floor. Just imagining the balloon touching your pelvic floor is enough to begin with.

10. Continue to expand the balloon on the inhale to the sides of your rib cage and to the back of your spine (step 3 in figure 5.5.2).

11. Lastly, fill your chest to full capacity. This should take about 6-10 seconds to do depending on your lung capacity and your level of experience with breathwork. (step 4 in figure 5.5.2).

12. On the exhalation, imagine the balloon contracting and letting air out from your chest and belly, pressing the belly up and in to exhale all of the air. Take about 6-10 seconds for the exhalation as well.

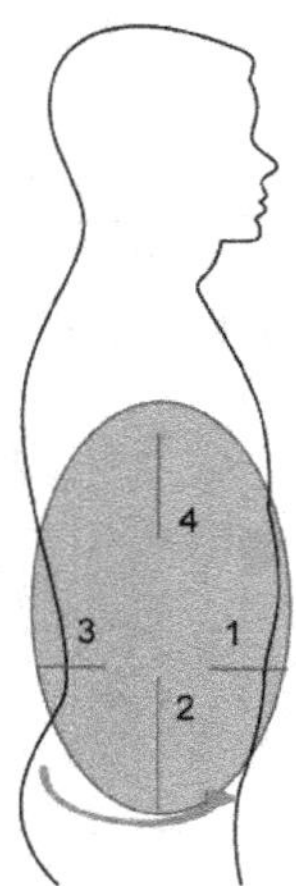

Figure 5.5.2

Comments:

This is the ultimate grounding and calming breath practice. It not only stimulates the vagus nerve, it increases heart rate variability and increases oxygen intake. Additionally, this technique has a calming effect on the survival brain, stimulating energy and blood flow to the gut, reproductive organs and pelvic area, which in yogic tradition is the seat of the root chakra (or First Chakra). The root chakra governs our survival need for "belongingness," or the feeling of being a part of a tribe.

Again, do not force your breath or your muscles. If you're feeling tightness in your lungs or in your lower organs that are below your rib cage or belly button, calmly tell these parts to relax before you continue. As with any new habit, it takes a few tries to get used to breathing and expanding your muscles this way.

Doing this simple breath exercise a couple of times a day or at the start of your yoga practice will go a long way towards strengthening and engaging your diaphragm. In turn, this exercise will gradually deepen your breath over time.

Caution: Overstimulating the Vagus Nerve

It's not easy to change your breathing habits and patterns overnight! The key is to never force it. Changing your breathing is like working a stiff muscle you haven't used in awhile — it will take time for your body to adapt to these techniques.

When doing these exercises, it's important that you don't overstimulate the vagus nerve. Did you know that overstimulating the vagus nerve is the most common cause of fainting? If you tremble or get queasy at the sight of blood or while getting a flu shot, you're not weak — you're experiencing what's known as "vagal syncope." That means that your body is responding to stress by overstimulating the vagus nerve, which causes your blood pressure and heart rate to drop.

During extreme "vagal syncope," blood flow is restricted to your brain and you lose conscious — that is, you faint. However, in most instances you just have to sit or lie down for symptoms to subside.

Relaxation Response and Longevity

Some recent studies have discovered a possible link between the relaxation response and overall longevity. In 2013, a team of researchers at Massachusetts General Hospital in Boston conducted an eight-week study on the effects of meditation and the relaxation response on the genes of volunteers who participated in the study.[8]

After eight weeks of performing these relaxation and meditation techniques daily — for only 10 to 20 minutes per day — the researchers analyzed any changes in the genes of the volunteers. [8] The results were fascinating. Clusters of important, beneficial genes had become more activated. These "boosted" genes showed an improvement in the efficiency of mitochondria and increased insulin production (which prevent the depletion of telomeres). This helps keep DNA stable, thus preventing cells from wearing out and aging.[8]

Some genes became less active, like a master gene that is known to trigger chronic inflammation. Sustained inflammation can lead to high blood pressure, heart disease, inflammatory bowel disease and some cancers.

This study illustrates just how beneficial practicing daily meditation and activating the relaxation response can be. Relaxing the body on a regular basis can change your body at the cellular level. That is a key ingredient of longevity and staying healthy as we age.

Practice Makes Perfect

Try all of the breathing techniques mentioned in this chapter and see which one you like best.

If you're a beginner, start with the basics, like the Anti-Stress Breathing Technique, Mindfulness Breath or Belly Breathing. Practice one exercise twice a day for for 21-30 days. Try starting with 3-5 minutes and work your way up to 10 minutes.

Other tips to get started:

- Schedule your breathing exercises into your smartphone. I like the "Timeless" iPhone app, which has a timer and calendar reminders. The

Timeless app allows you to set up a gentle reminder (it sounds like a gong) to remind you to do the exercises twice per day.

- Anchor your breathing exercise to an established habit or ritual, like going running or doing yoga. Most people remember to floss their teeth right after brushing their teeth, which then becomes a habit. Do the same thing with your breathing exercises by doing them before or after one of your regular habits or routines.

- Go easy on yourself! Don't beat yourself up if you miss a scheduled exercise — just practice your technique when you do find the time, even if you only practice for a few minutes. The important thing is that you do your exercises every day.

6

CHILL OUT & CALM DOWN

Conquer Anxiety with Muscle Relaxation

While in many ways the breath is a cornerstone of meditation, it's not the only way to reduce stress — muscle relaxation techniques can eliminate tension in the body, too, which helps us chill out and calm down in any situation.

Whether you realize it or not, you hold a lot of stress and tension in your body. Some of this is physical, like the tension in your shoulders that comes from being hunched over a computer for long periods of time. Your muscles also tense up as a fight-or-flight response (remember, this response evolved to as a way to protect ourselves from injury or pain when faced with danger).

In our hectic, nonstop world, we've become accustomed to feeling tense, especially in our neck, back and shoulders. However, having chronically tense muscles is not a normal condition. Rather, a lot of this tension comes from mental or emotional stress responses, which — whether we realize it or not — accumulate in our bodies over time.

One of the best ways to release tension in your body is through the use of muscle relaxation techniques. A specific form of these techniques is called Self-Directed Muscle Relaxation. (It's a slightly modified version of Autogenic relaxation training.) This technique involves relaxing targeted muscle groups while breathing slowly and evenly and mentally commanding your muscles to "Relax and let go" of tension. With practice, you can achieve deep physical relaxation and activate the relaxation response. This is the opposite of the stress response.

Benefits of Muscle Relaxation

- Reduces anxiety and panic attacks[1]
- Helps with insomnia and can help you fall asleep faster[2]
- Improves physical vitality, confidence and energy[3]
- Reduces stress throughout the day
- Aids in reducing performance anxiety, for both public speaking and sports performance[4]
- Activates the parasympathetic part of the autonomous nervous system, which improves digestion, promotes healthy bowel movements, lowers blood pressure, slows down the heart rate and boosts immunity[5]

How Self-Directed Muscle Relaxation Works

Self-Directed Muscle Relaxation (SDMR) is the practice of concentrating on a targeted muscle group and using mental and verbal commands to relax these muscles. In the early 1940s, SDMR was used by sports psychologists to help boxers and professional athletes deal with anxiety before a big match or game. Athletes who were trained in this technique showed a higher chance of winning than athletes who were not trained in relaxation techniques. Eventually, SDMR was also used in psychotherapy to help people deal with anxiety, depression and other mental health problems.

The opposite of muscle tension is relaxation. You have the power to train your body to relax in the face of stressful situations (instead of tensing up). Practicing relaxation techniques is all about learning to forget your past habits and making a relaxed state become your new normal.

When you think about it, learning always involves forgetting. With SDMR, you are forgetting your old habits and unconscious patterns and learning new skills to cope with stress, fear and anxiety.

Begin Small and Go Slow

When making big changes in our lives, it's perfectly normal to experience resistance. Have you ever tried to go on a diet and change how you eat overnight? Doesn't always work too well, does it?

Any time you try to adopt a new daily habit or get rid of an old one, you face resistance. Not only do you resist in your mind, you also experience physical resistance. This is why people swing from one extreme of dieting to the opposite, like going on a no-carb diet and then binging on carbs a few days later.

Resistance occurs because no one likes to be told what to do. Most people respond negatively to strong or direct suggestions: if someone tells us to stop smoking, drink less alcohol or eat less junk food, many of us get angry and rebel by not doing any of those things.

However, it's totally possible to learn new ways to change and to do so without resisting. By using gentler techniques like Self-Directed Muscle Relaxation, we shift the focus from resisting change to allowing change.

Allowing change to happen by letting go is much easier than fighting resistance to force change to happen. The exercises in this chapter will help you reprogram your mind — and your muscles — with a series of small suggestions. These exercises can lead to big changes in your stress levels and daily peace of mind.

6.1 Preparation Before Practicing Relaxation Exercises

When doing SDMR, preparation is the key to positive results. Here are some preparation tips:

1. Get a timer or timer app for your smartphone. I use a free timer app called "Timeless" (download from here: http://apple.co/2g5pAGa). Timeless has several alarm features that include interval alarms. It

can also record your relaxation progress over time with graphs and show you how much time you spend in your practice. It's only available for Apple iPhones and iPads.

2. Determine a location where you can practice without distraction. Ideally, you want to practice in the same place every day.

3. Figure out two times a day when you can practice your relaxation exercises. Stick to those times.

4. You can practice relaxation exercises sitting up or lying down flat or in a recliner chair or sofa. Initially, I recommend practicing lying down for the first two weeks because it's easier to relax when your body is in a horizontal position. You can transition to a sitting posture after the second week of practice.

5. I encourage you to make yourself as comfortable as possible, with pillows below your head, arms or legs if you are lying down.

6. If you choose a sitting posture for your practice, make sure you keep your spine straight without adding any strain or tension.

7. Each week, practice relaxing different muscle groups in the body. Remember: start small to create big changes with less resistance.

6.2 The 30 Day Transformation Program

Week 1: Relax Arms

During the first week, the focus is on relaxing your arms. Read the preparation instructions before starting (section 6.1).

Supporting Audio Link:

http://www.dchealthcoach.com/book/chapter-6

Time: 3 minutes twice a day

Keep your eyes closed during the practice.

1. Begin by doing the Anti-Stress Breathing Technique for 2 minutes (Chapter 5, exercise 5.1).
2. Relax the breath and breathe normally.
3. As you inhale through your nose, imagine your arms filling up with oxygen, starting from your fingertips, and traveling to your palms, forearms, biceps and triceps. The inhale should take 4-6 seconds.
4. As you exhale through your nose, mentally command the muscles around your arms to "Relax, let go, let go, let go…" This should take about 4-6 seconds.
5. Without trying to relax, just tell your arm muscles to relax on the exhale.
6. Repeat steps 3 through 5.

Comments:

The most important part of this exercise is to use the

verbal command: "Relax, let go, let go, let go…" in a slow, calm voice in your mind. That's it! Very simple and effective!

Week 2: Relax Legs and Arms

During the second week, we will work on relaxing your legs and arms. Read the preparation instructions before starting (section 6.1).

Supporting Audio Link:

http://www.dchealthcoach.com/book/chapter-6

Time: 5 minutes twice a day

Keep your eyes closed during the practice.

1. Begin by doing the Anti-Stress Breathing Technique for 2 minutes (Chapter 5, exercise 5.1).
2. Relax the breath and breathe normally.
3. For 1 minute, practice relaxing your arms (i.e., doing the exercise from the first week).
4. Next, shift your attention to your legs. As you inhale through your nose, imagine your legs filling up with oxygen, starting with your toes and moving up to your feet, calves, knees, thighs and buttocks. This inhalation should take 4-6 seconds.
5. As you exhale through your nose, mentally command your buttocks, thighs, knees, calves, and feet to

"Relax, let go, let go, let go…". This exhalation should take 4-6 seconds.

6. Without trying to relax, just tell your leg muscles to relax on the exhale.

7. Repeat steps 5 through 7.

Week 3: Back, Legs, and Arms

During the third week, we will work on relaxing your back, legs and arms. Read the preparation instructions before starting (section 6.1).

Supporting Audio Link:

http://www.dchealthcoach.com/book/chapter-6

Time: 10 minutes twice a day

Keep your eyes closed during the practice.

1. Begin by doing the Anti-Stress Breathing Technique for 2 minutes (Chapter 5, exercise 5.1).

2. Relax the breath and breathe normally.

3. For 2 minutes, practice relaxing your arms and legs (i.e., doing the exercises from the first and second weeks). Practice 1 minute for each muscle group.

4. Next, shift your attention to your back. As you inhale through your nose, imagine your back filling up with oxygen, starting from your lower back and moving

up to your mid back and upper back. This inhalation should take 4-6 seconds.

5. As you exhale through your nose, mentally command your upper back, mid back, and lower back to "Relax, let go, let go, let go…". This exhalation should take 4-6 seconds.

6. Without trying to relax, just tell your back muscles to relax on the exhale.

7. Repeat steps 5 through 7.

Week 4: Relax Chest and Belly, Back, Legs, and Arms

During the fourth week, we will work on relaxing your chest/belly, back, legs and arms. Read the preparation instructions before starting (section 6.1).

Supporting Audio Link:
http://www.dchealthcoach.com/book/chapter-6
Time: 15 minutes twice a day

1. Eyes are closed during the practice.

2. Begin by doing the Anti-Stress Breathing Technique for 2 minutes (Chapter 5, exercise 5.1).

3. Relax the breath and breathe normally.

4. For 3 minutes, practice relaxing your back, arms and legs. Practice 1 minute for each muscle group.

5. Next, shift your attention to your chest and belly. As you inhale through your nose, fill your belly and

chest with oxygen by expanding your belly first and then your chest. This inhalation should take 4-6 seconds.

6. As you exhale through your nose, mentally command your chest and belly and internal organs below your belly to "Relax, let go, let go, let go...". This exhalation should take 4-6 seconds.

7. Without trying to relax, just tell your back muscles to relax on the exhale.

8. Repeat steps 5 through 7.

Beyond Week Four: Graduate Program

You've made it all the way to Week 4 — congratulations! Continue with the same exercises and increase your practice time from 15 minutes to 20 minutes. Alternatively, add other muscle groups to the relaxation technique.

Week 5: Focus on letting go of the muscles around the neck and shoulders, along with the arms, chest, belly, legs and back. Time: 20 minutes.

Week 6: Focus on letting go of the muscles around the face, jaw, eye muscles and forehead along with the neck, shoulder, arms, chest, belly, legs and back. Time: 30 minutes.

What to Expect

When engaging in Self-Directed Muscle Relaxation, some people may notice muscle twitching in areas outside of the muscle group that's in focus. For example, you may feel twitching in your calves when you are telling your arms to "Let go," or you might feel twitching in random locations. This is normal. Much like your breath and heartbeat, your body has an autonomous way of self-organization and regulation. This is done automatically, without any conscious effort from you. The twitching you feel is part of this auto-function and is nothing to worry about.

Allow relaxation to happen naturally. As with any new practice, it takes time to adapt to change and make these habits a part of daily life. With a little patience, you will increase your awareness of how you respond to stress, and your old habits will become more obvious. Recognizing these habits and stressors is the first step in changing them.

Are We There Yet?

When doing these exercises, don't worry about whether or not you've achieved a deep level of relaxation yet. Stay positive and let relaxation occur at its own pace. When a distracting thought pops into your mind, don't dwell on it. Return to repeating "one." With practice, the relaxation response will come with little effort.

Practice this technique once or twice daily, but not within two hours after a meal — the digestive process can interfere with eliciting the relaxation response.

Don't *Try* to Relax

This sounds counterintuitive, but telling yourself "Try to relax!" does the opposite — it's a command that makes many of us tense up and makes us feel like we're doing something wrong. Telling yourself to "Relax, let go, let go, let go…" is a gentler stimulation, one that guides your muscles into relaxation whether you can feel that transformation or not.

Relax On Command

After two to three months of practicing this technique, you can use the "letting go" muscle relaxation exercise anywhere, anytime.

If you notice that you feel tense — or if you're an athlete about to play a sport — practice relaxing any part of your body for just a few minutes. Your body will call on the relaxation response instantly. This is the result of all those months of practice! By adding deep abdominal breathing to a muscle relaxation technique, your body will activate the relaxation response even quicker. Try it and play with how fast your body can relax in tense or stressful situations.

An Important Note About SDMR:

SDMR is an extremely safe technique that can be used by almost anyone, but there are a few exceptions:

- SDMR is not recommended for children under 5 years old.
- People with severe mental or emotional disorders should not attempt SDMR on their own, as it can lead to an increase in anxiety or restlessness. Someone with mental health disorders should be supervised by a professional instructor if they want to practice SDMR.
- If you are using SDMR to address a medical problem, talk to your doctor before getting started, as doing SDMR can affect your need for medication.

Practice Makes Perfect

Along with Self-Directed Muscle Relaxation (SDMR), there are other techniques that you can do to relieve tension in your muscles.

If you're already doing the breathing exercises discussed in Chapter 5, these muscle relaxation techniques are the next step in maintaining a more stress-free lifestyle.

By making muscle relaxation techniques a daily or weekly habit, you will notice the tightness and the tension in your body begin to evaporate. Over time and with practice, you can train your body to relax in a matter of seconds in response to just one command.

7

EMOTIONAL RELEASE: LETTING GO AND SURRENDERING

"The Cure for the Pain is in the Pain" -Rumi

We've all been told "Let it go!" with respect to something that's bugging us. Why is this so hard to do? I'm sure you've tried "letting it go" many times, yet you're still thinking about whatever "it" is no matter how hard you try not to.

"Letting go" isn't about forcing yourself to stop thinking about a particular issue or acting like you don't care about what's bothering you. To heal your body, you need to fully experience the negative emotions you've been holding onto and then release them. You have to let go of these negative thoughts and emotions that are no longer serving you. The act of "letting go" is a principal basis of self-healing.

Children practice letting go naturally. They experience a feeling — joy, anger, sadness — and then it passes. They move on. It's only when an adult or someone else tells us (as children or adults) that it's bad to express our emotions that we don't process these feelings.

As a kid, you were probably told to stop crying, or maybe you learned to bottle up your emotions on your own so as not to embarrass the adults around you. It's these past emotions that get stuck in our bodies. We can carry them around for years, long after the incident that triggered these feelings has passed.

When you let go of or relinquish negative emotions, you'll often experience a light or buoyant feeling. Letting go doesn't just help clear your mind — it can also release tension in your body and make you feel calmer, more relaxed and more at peace. Instead of telling yourself to just "let it go" with no result, we can practice the act of letting go on a recurring basis.

The exercises in this chapter will help you identify and experience your emotions without judging, analyzing, condemning or changing them. You can ride out your emotions as you would a storm instead of trying to stuff them down.

The result of this process is that old thinking patterns will no longer strongly trigger our emotions — instead, after releasing this powerful storm of emotions, a fresh wave of positive thoughts and feelings will bubble up to the surface.

The process of letting go isn't a one-time thing, but by engaging in these methods regularly, you will find that letting go gets easier over time.

Emotions Get Trapped in the Physical Body

A big part of emotional release is understanding that your emotions — even feelings you had years ago — get trapped in your body.

Your organs, tissues, skin, muscle and endocrine glands all have peptide receptors that can access and store emotional information.[1] Whether a feeling is a physical or and emotional one, it will translate to a peptide being released in some part of your body. This means that emotional memories are stored in many places in the body, not just your brain. You can access emotional memories anywhere in the peptide/receptor network and in a number of ways. [1]

Emotions that you hold in or never fully express are literally lodged in your body. These difficult, painful or uncomfortable emotions — which become trapped in your body after years of suppression — are exactly the emotions that need to be released. These emotions are trying to move up to the surface so that they can be released, made whole and healed.

Dr. Candace Pert, a well-known neuropharmacologist who has worked at the National Institutes of Health (NIH) and Georgetown University Medical Center, explains it best:

"Your body is your subconscious mind. Our physical body can be changed by the emotions we experience… Let the emotions bubble up. Let the chips fall where they may… The process of catharsis is not complete without saying things as the first step to experiencing things…To feel and understand means you have worked it all the way through. It has bubbled all the way to the surface. You're integrating at higher and higher levels in the body, bringing emotions into consciousness. Once integrated, the natural wisdom of the receptors will release interrupted healing and restorative and regenerative processes can take over."[1]

So in order to move forward in our lives, we need to practice emotional release.

Another way to think about it is this: the body doesn't have words to express itself, so it responds with physical sensations. Animals shake when they experience trauma or anxiety. Think of a dog that has been in a fight with another dog. Once the fight is over, both dogs will shake or tremble as a way to calm their nervous systems and quiet their fight-or-flight responses. This enables them to release any negative emotions about the fight and move on — without the physical memory of the situation.

Unlike other animals, humans don't naturally do this. Instead, we carry our stress, anxiety and trauma around with us. This leads to us using food, alcohol or other addictive substances (or behaviors) to soothe ourselves and quiet our emotional discomfort.

According to the Centers for Disease Control and Prevention (CDC), an estimated 85% of all diseases appear to have an emotional element. This is huge. Think of how much better everyone's health would be if we weren't constantly lugging all of our emotional baggage around in our bodies for decades on end!

Humans have a tendency to use our brains to forget, block or intellectualize our emotional memories, but the real focus should be on releasing the emotions stored in our bodies.

The good news is that there are ways to work through these emotions…and better yet, release them for once and for all. The exercises in this chapter will show you some great techniques for emotional release.

Note of Caution

Exercise caution when using these emotional release techniques on issues that may trigger re-traumatization. Avoid using these techniques on large traumas or distressing events like physical or sexual assault, combat/war zone, natural disaster, or terrorism, to name a few.

Please exercise discernment when using the emotional release techniques on small traumas like infidelity, divorce, starting a new job, legal trouble or financial worries to name a few. At times, processing smaller traumas could re-trigger or awaken larger traumas beneath the surface.

Seek the help of a therapist who specializes in trauma if you have any questions or concerns about your situation.

7.1 Emotional Release Technique #1: Allowing What Is

First, begin with a few mindful breaths to center yourself and bring yourself back to the present moment. You can practice the Mindfulness Breathing Exercise (exercise 5.2 in Chapter 5) or the Anti-Stress Breathing Technique (exercise 5.1 in Chapter 5) for 1-2 minutes.

Time: varies from 5 to 15 minutes

<u>Step 1: Being Present to What Is</u>
1. Identify an emotion or feeling that's bothering you.
2. As you identify this emotion, notice what's showing up for you. For example, you might feel some anxiety, but if you focus on your anxious thoughts,

your body might tense up or your breathing might speed up and become shallow.

3. Notice any associated feelings or any sensations in your body. Breathe and allow the sensations to be there without labeling them — just observe where they are in the body.

Step 2: Letting It Be

1. Your willingness to accept the sensations, thoughts, emotions or feelings may intensify them. That's OK. Keep breathing and allow the sensations to exist and bubble up. Give yourself and your body time to experience these sensations fully. Remember, resistance is causing you pain. Avoiding feeling those sensations allows those negative feelings to get stuck in our tissues, and that in turn has a negative impact on our health.

2. Give yourself and your body permission to experience the feelings fully by whispering "Yes" or "I consent." Gently and patiently let go of the guards you put up that have been protecting you from experiencing these feelings or sensations. We naturally (and sometimes unconsciously) avoid painful feelings through rational thinking or going outside of the body without feeling the pain. Gently

allowing ourselves a safe space to connect with our pain is the first step in healing ourselves.

3. If thoughts, judgments or stories distract you, draw your attention back to the breath and feeling any sensations that are present. We can't release these sensations by thinking our way through them, so every time your mind starts to analyze the sensations or you start to judge yourself for feeling them or thinking about the past or future, steer your attention back to your breath and where the sensations are in your body.

Comments:

There is no "right" or "wrong" experience — one of my clients once wanted to take a nap during an emotional release session. Taking a nap can be just as healing as letting go of old emotions. The "right" response is whatever is present and feels true for you at any given moment.

It's good to also let go of any expected outcomes or set goals. If we expect emotional release and relief as an outcome and don't get it, we could be setting ourselves up for disappointment when it doesn't happen. It's good to be non-attached to any particular outcome or direction your body wants to take during this process.

How long should you experience sensations? Each person's experience is different. Some people may take 5 minutes; others may take 10 to 15 minutes. It depends on how much you allow yourself to experience the feeling/sensations.

Caution: if you are facing traumatic experiences or feelings, please seek professional advice. Use your best judgment as to whether or not you want to revisit those traumatic experiences. It's important not to retraumatize yourself with painful experiences and to see a professional if you need to help dealing with intense or difficult emotions.

Eventually, given enough time, you'll ride out your feelings the way you would a storm. Everyone's experience is unique. Some people weep; others fall asleep. Anger and rage may surface. The key is to allow whatever shows up to show up and to let yourself ride it out (figure 7.1.1).

This emotional awareness technique can be used in any place or situation. You can even use it at the end of or during the relaxation and breathing exercises from the previous chapters.

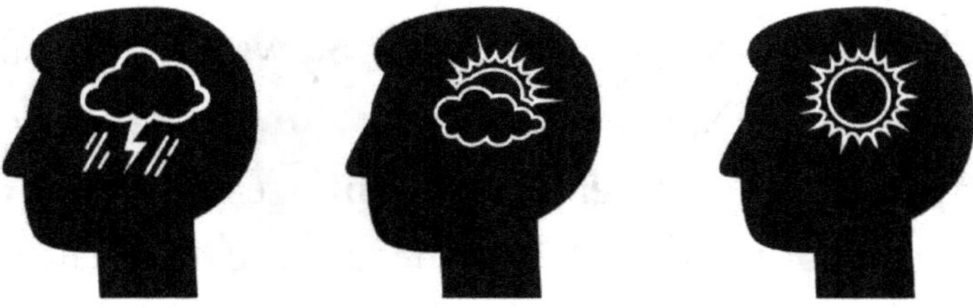

Figure 7.1.1

7.2 Emotional Release Technique #2: Diving Deep

The following emotional release technique is borrowed from various disciplines and counseling techniques, including somatic psychology, embodiment and co-counseling. I have developed and refined this technique through my coaching practice and through my personal emotional release work.

First, begin with a few mindful breaths to center yourself and bring yourself back to the present moment.

You can use the Mindfulness Breathing Exercise (exercise 5.2 in Chapter 5) or the Anti-Stress Breathing Technique (exercise 5.1 in Chapter 5) for 2 minutes.

Preparation

1. Find a place where you can practice this technique privately and without distraction.
2. Give yourself permission to be vulnerable and know that it's safe to feel whatever feelings and sensations that may surface during this process.
3. Know that you can stop any time whenever you feel uncomfortable.
4. Practice non-attachment to the outcome. The goal is not to experience emotional release all at once — sometimes your body just wants to eat or sleep, and that in and of itself is healing enough. At the same time, using this technique is an open invitation for your subconscious to release some of its baggage. This baggage may show up as an emotional release or feeling like you need a hug or want to fall asleep. However you and your body respond to emotional release is right for you.

Time: 10 - 15 minutes

Step 1: Identify the Limiting Belief or Stressor

1. Identify something that's bothering you at the moment (e.g., you're anxious about the future or fearful of losing your job). This could also be a limiting or negative belief about yourself ("I'm not good enough," "I'm not worthy").

2. In one short sentence or phrase, describe what's bothering you. For example, you could identify with "I am so stressed out right now!". As you say that to yourself, your body might let out a sigh. Then you may notice your belly tensing up.

3. Repeat the phrase: "I'm so stressed out" (or whatever phrase that's true right now). As you do so, direct the statement down to your belly area, which is where many of us hold most of our anxiety and stress.

4. There is a common saying: "The energy flows where our attention goes." By voicing our feelings aloud and directing our statements to the belly, we are inviting your subconscious to open up to healing and unlocking trapped emotions.

Step 2: Recognize the Feelings

1. Begin to notice whatever emotions, feelings, thoughts or sensations these phrases bring up.

2. For example, "I'm feeling unworthy" can trigger sadness. From a scale of 1-10, notice how strong that

feeling is. If it's a 5 or higher, continue to use that phrase as a starting point.

3. The key to this technique is to identify phrases that have a strong emotional trigger. As you work with those phrases, you will continue to dive deeper into your subconscious and unlock old emotions that have been buried for many years. You may also reveal some limiting core beliefs.

4. As you continue to repeat the phrase to yourself, directing your voice down to your gut and belly area, the emotions or feelings may intensify.

Step 3: Surrender and Let Go

1. Stay with your body and the sensations that arise from this process.

2. Your willingness to accept the sensations, thoughts, emotions or feelings may intensify them. That's OK. Keep breathing and allow the sensations to exist and bubble up. Give yourself and your body the time to experience those sensations fully. Your resistance is what's causing you pain.

3. Allow your body to release itself in the form of tears, anger or an outcry. However your body chooses to express the pain is right the response and right mode of healing.

4. Continue repeating the phrase until it doesn't trigger an emotional response or until the emotional scale is below a 4 or 3. This may take several minutes or up to 15 minutes.

5. You will get to a point where you no longer feel those feelings, or at least not as strongly as before. If you repeat the phrase, at this point, it will no longer have power over you.

6. At the end of this process, one may experience a feeling of buoyancy, lightness and even joy. One of my clients wanted to take a nap because that what his body wanted at the time. Another client experienced peace and stillness within 5 minutes after releasing her fear and anxiety.

Comments:

A good way to think about this technique is to use the analogy of fishing: imagine that the phrases you say and your voice are the hook and line to catch the big fishes (your old emotional baggage). These big fishes/your emotional baggage hide at the bottom of the ocean (your subconscious).

When we let the fishing line (your voice) travel deep into the water (belly/gut area), we may catch a few small fishes. If we're lucky, we may even get a very big one. Once we have a catch (the emotions, sensations or feelings in the body), we reel it up to the surface and bring it to light (expressing the emotions/feelings). As we continue with the emotional release by repeating the triggering phrase, we free up the stored and stuck energy that no longer serves us. We end up freeing space and making room for other, healthier emotions.

Step 4: Diving Deeper (Optional)

Some people find many benefits when using the above techniques, and those benefits may be enough. If you would like to go deeper with this process and uncover your core limiting beliefs, however, then you can add the following steps to the above process:

1. Continue to repeat the phrases that have strong triggers (from Step 3: Letting Go and Surrender).
2. Continue to release in whatever way your body expresses itself.
3. As you repeat the phrase and simultaneously experience release, other phrases or limiting beliefs may show up. Switch to a new phrase if you feel it has a strong emotional pull that will allow you to release even more — let "I'm not good enough" to turn into "I'm not loved," for example.
4. Continue to release and repeat the phrase until you experience a shift in emotions towards a lighter emotion. This may take several minutes.

5. Once you have experienced a shift, you can then ask your body, "What is the message here?" "What are you trying to tell me?" Listen closely — the first answer is usually the correct answer. Try not to consciously think of a solution; rather, become the solution by allowing the answer to bubble up naturally. This is what's called "an inner knowing."

6. If you receive an answer during this step, repeat the answer to yourself and notice how you feel when you say it to yourself. It could be a new belief about yourself, a positive message or a new perception you hadn't had before.

7. You may start to notice shifts in your emotions from a dense and tight space to an expanded and light space.

8. Continue to repeat the new positive phrase.

9. At some point, ask your body "Is there anything else you want me to know?" or "How can I support you?"

10. Listen patiently and make note of it later, after you've completed the process.

11. Continue to notice the shifts in energy and sensations in your body. Notice the way you're breathing or holding your posture. Acknowledge that you just went through a lot of emotional release and that you did great.

<u>**Wrapping Up: Get Grounded**</u>

One way to clear up some of the energy from our release is to do one of these grounding and clearing exercises:

1. Go outside in the sun barefoot and sit on the grass. Allow your feet to touch the ground.
2. Splash your hands, arms, face and back of the neck with cold water.
3. Shake off the energy by vigorously shaking your hands and arms in front of you, much like a dog shakes its body after a good walk.
4. Talk to a friend afterward. You can share what you experienced or just connect with them and catch up.

Comments:

I want to emphasize that everyone's experience at the end of the process is different. There is no one-size-fits all model for emotional release…although, more often than not, a lighter emotion is a good indication that the process worked. It is important to not to be attached to the outcome — if you didn't experience joy at the end of your release, that it doesn't mean it didn't work. You might feel disappointed if you don't experience joy every time after doing an emotional release technique, but joy is not always the goal of this process. If you allow your uniqueness to unfold before you and you cherish the messages that your intelligence presents to you, then we all can come to a place where we are more fully integrated and whole beings.

A cautionary note: in doing these emotional release techniques, I do not suggest working with situations like a divorce or a death in the family, issues that can bring up very intense emotions. According to David Hawkins, with these kinds of difficult situations, it's best to indulge in some avoidance or coping mechanisms and revisit them with a professional later. Hawkins suggests breaking up those emotions into chunks and working with them individually — and over time — instead of trying to tackle all of your emotions at once. Also, it's best to seek professional advice when dealing with traumatic experiences.

Client's Breakthrough with Emotional Release

"Working with Vincent and his emotional release technique, I was able to confront a buried reality: that I had given up my voice in my marriage and that in turn I had given up on myself. For many years, I had bottled up insecurity and powerlessness around my role in my marriage. I was less and less myself around my wife whom I love dearly, but voiceless in expressing my emotional needs and a longing for spirituality. I had ceded control of nearly all aspects of my life both daily and long term.

Initially, it was very scary and also embarrassing to face my emotions. With Vincent's gentle guidance, I gave voice to my shadows and allowed myself to be heard, expressed and acknowledged. I couldn't believe how painful it was to feel the emotions and how long I've been ignoring them. He guided me down into very dark and cold place where I saw myself slowly dying inside. I was harboring a hopeless mantra: "I'm dying, it's over for me, I have nothing left." I connected with that pain, that wounded inner child, and I gave it a voice. I gave myself permission to feel the pain and suffering. He helped me open up a wound that had long been buried deep.

After two short sessions, Vincent gave me the tool and insights on how to connect and release my emotions safely without shame. He helped me create a new relationship with my body and my inner child. I have slowly regained power in self-care and starting to carve out time in my schedule for activities that are fulfilling for me. I started rock climbing and also took a look at my career and made much needed changes. I'm taking baby steps to improve my relationship with my wife, and express more openly with her. I've connected with a support group for men and began weekly sessions where I can freely express my emotions without judgement. I'm now coming from a newly opened and reclaimed place inside, and I'm finally climbing." Brian Z.

Letting Go Before Bedtime

One of the best times to practice emotional release is before going to bed.

Any negative feelings, stresses and anxieties that arose during the day — like an argument you had with your spouse or partner, a looming work deadline or stress at home, in the office or at school — can keep you tossing and turning in bed for hours before you eventually fall asleep.

A better bedtime routine is to practice the "letting go" technique along with the deep relaxation exercises from Chapter 2 and diaphragmatic breathing from Chapter 1 before you go to sleep. These three exercises can greatly reduce insomnia and make for a more restful, restorative sleep every night.

Journaling is another extremely beneficial bedtime ritual. Journaling can be its own emotional release, allowing you to get your worries, thoughts and feelings down on paper rather than holding them in and letting them build up and fester. Multiple studies have shown that journaling can help you process and release some negative emotions.

8

PUTTING IT ALL TOGETHER

The 21-Day Challenge and Beyond

Up until this point, every chapter has included several great de-stressing and relaxation tools that you can use any time, anywhere. All of these exercises only a take a few minutes to do and can easily be added to your daily routine.

This chapter is about putting it all together: combining everything you've learned in the previous chapters and stacking them to get the best results. I highly recommend practicing some of the exercises in the previous chapter before diving into the techniques and activities in this chapter, especially if you are a beginner or are new to breathworks.

Setting the Tone

Mornings can be a stressful time. Most of us wake up to an alarm clock — which immediately puts you in fight-or-flight mode and gets your cortisol and adrenaline pumping before you even get out of bed!

Many of us are so rushed in the morning that we skip breakfast, down a large cup of coffee and sprint out the door — which revs up the adrenaline and cortisol hormones even more. After you leave the house, you have to deal with bumper to bumper traffic or hurry to catch your bus or train. Going through this everyday makes being stressed out a daily routine. If you're like most people, mornings are a bitch.

But guess what? It doesn't have to be this way. You can establish a much more relaxing routine — which will set the tone for the rest of your day. What you do in the morning has a huge effect on how you move through the day.

Wouldn't you rather wake up well-rested, energized and ready to take the day by storm, instead of opening your eyes and immediately feeling a wave of stress-induced panic? My morning routine helps me go about my day in a relaxed state with ease. In the mornings, if I do some meditative exercises — like yoga or deep breathing — I feel emotionally and mentally centered for several hours afterward. It's possible for you to feel this way everyday too.

When we are calm and relaxed, we are less reactive to stressful circumstances — like sitting in traffic — that we often have little control over. If we can reduce the daily stress in your lives, even by just a little bit, this gives us more energy and the space spend our time in more meaningful ways and do the things that matter to us. Diminishing our daily stressors also results in better health overall, for both our minds and our bodies.

8.1 The 21-Day Total Transformation Challenge (Beginners)

<u>Week 1 Challenge: The Morning Experiment</u>
Week one of the 21-day challenge focuses on practicing some of the exercises in the book and noticing how they affect your mood and energy throughout the day.

Time: 5-10 minutes

For the First 3 Days:
1. Do the Seated Forward Bend exercise in Chapter 4, exercise 4.7. Do this for 2-5 minutes, breathing deeply in and out through your nose while holding the forward bend pose.
2. Practice the Belly Breath for 3-5 minutes every day in the morning at the same time. Ideally, you would do this before breakfast but after you've had a glass of water, brushed your teeth and finished your other daily morning routines. Or you can do any of the other breathing techniques instead as long as you stick to whatever you choose and do it daily.

On Days 4 through 7:
3. On Day 4, skip the forward bend and breathing exercises and go back to your normal morning routine. Notice how you feel throughout the

morning and rest of the day. In the evening, write down any changes you experienced.

4. On Days 5 through 7, continue the challenge by repeating steps 1 and 2 from above.

Week 2 Challenge: Midday Check-In and Reset

Stress can throw us off at any time during the day. This happens to even the most experienced meditators. The key is to recognize when we are off-center and to know that we have the tools to re-center ourselves.

During this week, we will continue the morning routine from Phase One and add in a midday check-in. Midday could between 1 to 3 p.m. or whenever you're feeling especially stressed-out and un-centered.

Time: 5 minutes

1. Find a space in your office or at home where you can do the Standing Inversion: Forward Bend in chapter 4, exercise 4.2.

2. Inhale deeply through your mouth and exhale complete out through your nose for 2-3 minutes when you are in the Forward Bend.

3. When the 3 minutes are up, slowly return to standing upright.

4. End with the Anti-Stress Breathing Technique from chapter 5, exercise 5.1. Practice the breathwork with your eyes closed for 2 minutes.

Week 3 Challenge: Evening Routine

It's not uncommon for stress to cause many of us to make poor decisions, especially when it comes to diet and lifestyle choices. One of my past clients, Susan, had a bad habit of eating whatever was in the fridge at home after a stressful workday. Before she started working with me, Susan kept lots of unhealthy foods and junk foods stocked in the fridge. Every time she engaged in stress eating, Susan would gain weight. She really wanted to stop her stressful eating patterns from getting out of control.

In addition to always keeping healthy options in the fridge, I suggested that Susan do some meditation or breathing exercises as soon as she got home. She did, and this had a big impact on her poor eating habits — she saw positive results right away. Susan no longer had to deal with feeling guilty about eating junk food, plus she found it easier to eat healthy and make better choices.

Even when we have the best intentions, stress can make it difficult for us to make healthy choices. Our body is designed to numb out pain and seek pleasure. Our body wants to eat that piece of cheesecake because it gives us a pleasurable sensation even though in our minds we know that eating foods full of sugar isn't good for us.

Much like a morning routine, an evening relaxation routine not only helps us unwind, it also helps us reconnect with our wiser and deeper inner self. This inner reconnection reminds us of what's important. When we are acting from a place of calmness and peace, our decisions to make healthy lifestyle and food choices are effortless. We are no longer powerless victims of our body's natural instincts — instead, we can gently guide ourselves to making better, healthier diet choices and improving our lifestyle habits.

The Evening Routine:

Time 3-5 minutes

1. If you have time, take a quick shower as soon as you get home. Otherwise, splash your face, eyes and neck (front and back) with cold water. Wet your arms and wrists as well.

2. Dry off and literally shake out the stress of the day from your hands and arms, shaking and twisting your wrist and arms rigorously up and down and side to side.

3. Find a spot in your house to do your evening relaxation routine (ideally the same place you did your morning routine).

4. With your eyes closed, do the Anti-Stress Breathing Technique (chapter 5, exercise 5.1) for 2 minutes.

5. Relax and let go: with your eyes closed, relax different parts of your body by mentally telling your muscles relax on command (see chapter 7). Start from your legs and tell your leg muscles to "Relax, and let go, let go, let go…" Do this 2 to 3 times, and then move attention to your back muscles, then slowly transition to your arms, chest, belly, neck, shoulder, face, eyes, and forehead. With each body part, spend about 2 to 3 times telling it to "Relax and let go, let go, let go…" Have a relaxed breath. Time: 5 minutes.

6. Finally, after the relaxation exercise, notice anything that's showing up for you in the moment. It could be sensations in the body—you're feeling more relaxed or centered. You may notice some stuck or unprocessed emotions from the day. If you want to process those emotions, you can practice the "letting go" emotional release technique in chapter 7,

exercise 7.1 for 5-10 minutes until the stressor or emotions have moved through your system. Journaling is also a great tool as well.

Congratulations!

Congrats on making it through your first 21 days of relaxation and deep breathing exercises! If you did these exercises every day you likely have noticed the following:

- Heightened awareness of where you hold tension in your body
- Increased lung capacity (since your body is used to the deep breathing)
- Increased vitality and energy
- Feeling more centered and calm throughout the day
- Reacting less
- Increased awareness of how people and circumstances triggers your mood and emotions.

If you didn't experience of any of those, that's totally fine, too — you probably experienced other positive outcomes that are not on this list.

The Total Reboot

Remember the last time your computer froze? You were probably running too many programs at the same time. When this happens, most of us grunt with annoyance, pound the keys for a few minutes and then try to reboot the computer.

Our minds and our bodies can get overwhelmed and freeze up as well. When our "monkey mind" is entertaining too many thoughts at once or tackling too many problems in our heads, one of our natural instincts is to retreat and avoid what's really going on. We freeze up. We seek out things that give us instant gratification, like junk food or alcohol. We distract ourselves as a way of not dealing with our real problems.

These avoidance strategies work for a short period of time, but as we keep procrastinating, our mental stress builds up, leading to burnout and other damaging effects on our physical bodies. During periods of chronic stress, our nervous and immune systems suffer and our health is negatively affected.

The best way to combat a total physical, mental or emotional shutdown is to perform a daily reboot. Hitting the restart button — on both your body and your brain — should be a part of everyone's daily stress management and anti-burnout plan.

This Brain Belly Balance exercise will help you do a mental, physical and emotional energy reboot in as little as 5 minutes.

8.2 Brain-Belly-Balance Exercise (Intermediate)

Time: 5 minutes

1. Start with doing the March in Place or Cross Crawl (chapter 4, exercise 4.14) for 30 seconds, as a way to synchronize the left and right hemispheres of the brain.
2. Follow this with the Standing Inversion: Forward Bend (chapter 4, exercise 4.2) for 1 minute.
3. Rub your ears for 30 seconds. This increases circulation throughout your body.
4. While sitting or lying down, practice the 1 Minute Breathing Exercise (chapter 5, exercise 5.4).

Freedom from Blocks and Procrastinations

We have all experienced procrastination, whether it's in the form of writer's block or avoiding simple chores like doing the laundry, washing the dishes or taking out the trash. We experience many other forms of resistance, too. Most of the time, this starts with an emotional resistance or blockage — we tell ourselves "It's too hard" or "I don't want to do this." These thoughts create a cascade of negative feelings that freeze us in our tracks.

But if you look at the chore you're resisting (e.g., taking out the trash), that particular activity is no different from any other task. When we label an activity as "hard" or put it in the "I don't enjoy doing this" category, we build up even more resistance to the task itself. However, if we look at "hard" tasks we don't want to do and compare them with tasks we don't mind doing, we find that they often require the same amount of time and effort. In many instances, our feelings about the task make it more difficult and increase our resistance to do these chores.

The following exercises (which combine what you've learned in previous chapters) can be extremely helpful for unblocking your mind and releasing resistance.

8.3 Unblock Procrastination Exercise

1. Focus on the task or chore that you're procrastinating or resisting. Recognize that you don't enjoy doing this activity.

2. Practice the first emotional release technique from Chapter 8 (exercise 8.1). Recognize the emotions that are showing up for you when you practice this technique. Notice the ways that your body wants to express its resistance. Any response is appropriate: sighing, anger, stretching, beating the couch, etc. Whatever shows up for you is the right response.

3. You can also express to yourself by vocalizing why you don't enjoy doing the task, like saying "It's too damn hard." Take a moment to be with any feelings or sensations in your body as you express this statement several times.

4. Once those feelings or sensations pass (and they usually do), then try the following exercises from previous chapters to get you centered and reconnected with your body.

    a. Ear Rubbing technique from Chapter 4, exercise 4.1

    b. Do the 1-Minute Breath exercise on Chapter 5, exercise 5.4.

    c. Practice the Brain Workout exercises in Chapter 4 of Getting Unstuck: Choose either the cross crawl (exercise 4.4) or eye focusing exercise (exercise 4.6).

5. Now go back to the task at hand. Recognize that every task is a series of small steps or actions. Try writing down all of the steps involved, no matter

how small they are. When you write down the steps, you can also visualize yourself doing the task relaxed and at ease. Remind yourself that in the grand scheme of life, each of these tiny steps isn't that big of a deal…unless you attach meaning to it.

6. Celebrate your progress! You've unblocked a block! Next time you experience resistance, repeat steps 1 through 5. Over time, all of your "hard" tasks will become easier and easier to do.

Comments:

When it comes to completing bigger tasks or projects that will take a significant amount of time, you might feel a huge amount of emotional resistance at first. This could be because your end goal seems (or feels) so far away when you're at the very beginning of the process. Instead of resisting or avoiding this pain, let your emotions happen. For some of us, our natural inclination is to freeze up and avoid these negative feelings. However, if you keep practicing these unblocking exercises, it becomes easier to release resistance and focus on getting the project done — your old habit of procrastination will diminish, and your new habit of unblocking and letting go will take its place.

9

THE JOURNEY CONTINUES

*"A Journey of a Thousand Miles Begins with
a Single Step" – Lao Tsu*

By practicing the exercises and techniques in this book,
you've made a giant leap forward onto the path of being
mindful and living a more centered, peaceful existence.
When you make daily commitments to work on staying
in the moment, reduce stress, let go and release

emotional baggage, the benefits extend far beyond feeling more relaxed and at ease on a regular basis.

As you continue to do these breathing and relaxation exercises and make them daily habits, my hope for you is that you will also experience immense growth and changes in your spiritual and emotional well-being. By focusing on your breath, you are actually opening yourself up to an inner wisdom that resides in all of us, a wisdom that speaks to us if we take the time to listen.

So many books about meditation and mindfulness make it seem like all of this stuff should be hard...but it doesn't have to be. The philosophy behind all of the techniques in Breathe, Repeat is that you don't have to be a seasoned expert or a practiced yogi to get the full benefits of these exercises. By simply making an effort to incorporate these exercises into your daily routine, you are well on your way to seeing positive results: physically, mentally and emotionally.

Taking better care of yourself and improving your health is an investment, one whose rewards greatly increase over time. Even after finishing Breathe, Repeat and completing the 21-Day Total Transformation Challenge, your journey is far from over. As you go deeper with each exercise and technique, you will uncover new truths and discoveries within yourself and you will unearth more emotional blockages that need to be released.

As you continue on your path to mindfulness, use this book as a guidepost for daily practice and reflection. Keep it handy and refer to it often. Use Breathe, Repeat as a daily mantra and reminder to yourself that living a balanced and relaxed lifestyle doesn't cost anything and is available to you any time, anywhere. Don't forget to share the techniques you've learned with others.

Share your own story, too. No one wants to live a life of chronic stress and chaos, but many people just don't know how or where to begin. You can be an inspiration to others!

And remember, the first step is easy:
Just breathe and repeat.

REFERENCES

Chapter 3

1. McClatchy. "Studies Show Stress Can Reshape the Brain." The Guardian, Guardian News and Media, 19 Nov. 2008, www.theguardian.com/science/2008/nov/19/brain-stress-research-reshape.

Chapter 4,

1. Streeter, Chris C., et al. "Yoga Asana Sessions Increase Brain GABA Levels: A Pilot Study." THE JOURNAL OF ALTERNATIVE AND COMPLEMENTARY MEDICINE, vol. 13, no. 4, 2007, pp. 419–426., doi:10.1089/acm.2007.6338.

Chapter 5, Breathe Like Your Life Depends On It

1. Perkins, A. (1994). Savings money by reducing stress. Harvard Business Review. 72(6):12.
2. "The Relaxation Response." Wikipedia, Wikimedia Foundation, 22 Sept. 2017, en.wikipedia.org/wiki/The_Relaxation_Response.
3. Killingsworth, M A, and D T Gilbert. "A Wandering Mind Is an Unhappy Mind." Science (New York, N.Y.)., U.S. National Library of Medicine, 12 Nov. 2010, www.ncbi.nlm.nih.gov/pubmed/21071660.
4. Wang, SZ, et al. "Effect of Slow Abdominal Breathing Combined with Biofeedback on Blood Pressure and Heart Rate Variability in Prehypertension." PubMed, The Journal of Alternative and Complementary Medicine, Oct.

2010,doi:10.1089/acm.2009.0577 www.ncbi.nlm.nih.gov/pubmed/20954960.

5. Bergland, Christopher. "Vagus Nerve Stimulation Dramatically Reduces Inflammation." Psychology Today, Sussex Publishers, 6 July 2016, www.psychologytoday.com/blog/the-athletes-way/201607/vagus-nerve-stimulation-dramatically-reduces-inflammation.

6. Adelson, Rachel. "Stimulating the Vagus Nerve: Memories Are Made of This." Monitor on Psychology, American Psychological Association, Apr. 2004, www.apa.org/monitor/apr04/vagus.aspx.

7. Lehrer, Paul M., and Richard Gevirtz. "Heart Rate Variability Biofeedback: How and Why Does It Work?" Frontiers, Frontiers, 27 June 2014, www.frontiersin.org/articles/10.3389/fpsyg.2014.00756/full.

8. Coghlan, Andy. "Meditation Boosts Genes That Promote Good Health." New Scientist, May 2013, www.newscientist.com/article/dn23480-meditation-boosts-genes-that-promote-good-health/.

Chapter 6

1. Manzoni, Gian Mauro, et al. "Relaxation Training for Anxiety: a Ten-Years Systematic Review with Meta-Analysis." BMC

2. Psychiatry, BioMed Central, 2008, www.ncbi.nlm.nih.gov/pmc/articles/PMC2427027/.

3. Bowden, A, et al. "Autogenic Training as a Behavioural Approach to Insomnia: a Prospective Cohort Study." Primary Health Care Research & Development., U.S. National Library of Medicine, Apr. 2012, www.ncbi.nlm.nih.gov/pubmed/21787446.

4. Ortigosa-Márquez, J.M., et al. "Effects of Autogenic Training on Lung Capacity, Competitive Anxiety and Subjective Vitality."

Biomedical Research, Allied Academies, 5 Oct. 2014, www.alliedacademies.org/articles/effects-of-autogenic-training-on-lung-capacity-competitive-anxiety-andsubjective-vitality.html.

5. Kornspan, Alan S., and Mary J. MacCracken. "Psychology Applied to Sport in the 1940s: The Work of Dorothy Hazeltine Yates." The Sport Psychologist, vol. 15, 2001, pp. 342–345., www.humankinetics.com/AcuCustom/Sitename/Documents/DocumentItem/1873.pdf.

Chapter 7

1. Pert, Candace B. Molecules of Emotion: Why You Feel the Way You Feel. Scribner, 2003.

2. Perkins, A. (1994). Savings money by reducing stress. Harvard Business Review. 72(6):1

ABOUT THE AUTHOR

Vincent Hu is a Washingtonian native of over 25 years. He is a graduate of the Institute for Integrative Nutrition® in New York, accredited with the American Association of Drugless Practitioners, and certified as a Health Counselor in Integrative Nutrition® through Columbia University's Teacher's College.

Vincent has studied with master teachers in the health field & is trained in modern health counseling, eastern & western nutrition philosophies & uses nutrition, yoga & meditation for therapeutic improvement. His experience as a professional yoga instructor & student of meditation adds a depth to his work that attunes to the whole person. With over 15 years experience in the corporate world, he understands the challenges of staying healthy while pursuing a career. This familiarity enables Vincent to gently guide his clients to release self-sabotaging behaviors with a unique blend of nutrition coaching & stress relieving strategies.

http://www.dchealthcoach.com

ACKNOWLEDGEMENT

Thank you, divine spirit mystery of the universe, for letting there be beaches, sunshine, Hong Kong latte, Erewhon, and gluten-free quinoa bread. Owen Kono Bee, the Astrologer for the Stars and White Pugs. Rosanna Turner, Lisa Howard, and Jason Anscomb. Dawn Hoffman and #26. Sakib and his big heart. Kayleigh for her generosity. Aga my accountability partner.